D1015687

VENUS ON FIRE
MARS ON ICE

VENUS
ON FIRE
MARS ON ICE

HORMONAL BALANCE—THE KEY
TO LIFE, LOVE, AND ENERGY

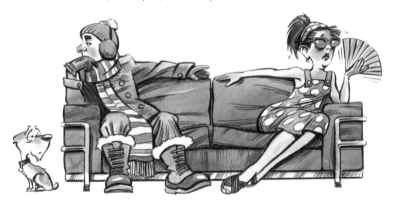

FROM THE AUTHOR OF THE #1 BESTSELLER
MEN ARE FROM MARS, WOMEN ARE FROM VENUS

JOHN GRAY, Ph.D.

WITH FOREWORD BY HYLA CASS, M.D.

VENUS ON FIRE MARS ON ICE

 Mind Publishing

For information contact:
Mind Publishing
PO Box 57555
1031 Burnette Ave.
Coquitlam, BC, V3K 1E0

www.mindpublishing.com

info@mindpublishing.com

ISBN 978-0-9782797-3-8
Printed in Canada

Design: FWH Creative

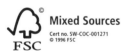 **Mixed Sources**
Cert no. SW-COC-001271
© 1996 FSC
FSC

This book is printed using vegetable-based inks on FSC certified paper, which is chlorine free, old growth free, harvested using sustainable forest practices, and 100% biodegradable.

ACKNOWLEDGMENTS

I thank my wife, Bonnie, for sharing the journey of developing this book with me. For 25 years she has been a great teacher as well as my biggest fan. She is a tremendous source of insight and her capacity to love is a great inspiration. I thank her for expanding my ability to understand and honor the female point of view. This perspective has not only enriched our life together but also provides the foundation for the many insights in this book.

I thank our three daughters, Shannon and her husband Jon, Juliet and her husband Dan, and Lauren, for their continuous love and support. Our many conversations have definitely enriched my perspective on what it means to be a young woman today. The love we share and the many challenges they have each overcome have helped anchor the many practical ideas in Venus on Fire Mars on Ice. I also thank our grandchildren, Sophia Rose, Bo Oliver and Bradyn James for the new joy and delight they have brought to our family.

I thank my staff and support team, Bonnie Gray, Katie Bushnell, Marci Wynne, Gary Thompson, Renee DeBruin, Susan Burns, Rich Bernstein, Jeff Owens, Dean W. Levin, Elley Coren, Sherrie Nattrass, and Russ and Carol Burns, for their consistent support and hard work in organizing and producing my talks, seminars, columns, internet TV and radio show, nutritional product development and distribution, MarsVenus.com website, AskMarsVenus.com telephone coaching, MarsVenusDating.com and our monthly Mars Venus Wellness Retreats. For a small group of people you do a lot.

I want to say a special thanks to Dean W. Levin for his loyalty and strategic marketing expertise which greatly supports and facilitates translating my ideas and concepts into active Mars Venus ventures. I thank Rich Bernstein, Jim Taylor and Melodie Tucker for their support in creating and sustaining the Mars Venus Executive Coaching training program which is active around the world. Because of their continuous support, our Mars Venus Executive coaches experience increasing success. I also want to thank my editorial staff, Martin and Josie Brown, at the MarsVenusLiving. com online magazine and my daughter Lauren Gray for her brilliant relationship column Guys Are From Mars, Chicks Are From Venus. In addition, I want to thank the many Mars Venus Counselors for their dedication to bringing these insights to their clients. I also want to thank the hundreds of supportive people who help our team bring this message to the world.

The ideas in this book are certainly inspired by my own personal experiences in creating a loving relationship and in helping others do the same but without the thousands of people who have generously shared their insights, experiences and research it could never have been so rich. Each page has some jewel of wisdom that I have cherished in hearing and I know you, the reader, will as well. To gather these ideas, it has taken a team of dedicated health, happiness and relationship teachers, writers, coaches, researchers, therapists, doctors, nurses, patients and seminar participants over thirty years to refine and develop. Much of this work in developing the new ideas for Venus on Fire Mars on Ice was done through special gatherings and seminars at the Mars Venus Wellness Center in Northern California over the past eight years. I thank my parents, Virginia and David Gray, for all their love and support, and Lucille Brixey, who was always like a second mother to me. Although they are no longer here, their love and encouragement continue to surround and bless me.

This book is dedicated
with deepest love and affection

to my wife, Bonnie Gray, and our three daughters
Lauren, Juliet and Shannon.
Their love has supported me to be the best I can be,
and to share with others what we have
learned together as a family.

FOREWORD

BY HYLA CASS, M.D.

Science has now proven what we have always instinctively known: that the mind and body are inseparably linked. Now in his new book, John Gray explains how our minds and moods are affected by our hormones, and how hormonal balance is key to successful relationships and joyful living.

John has helped millions of couples with their relationships by unraveling their complicated feelings, and will now address, using his simple but enlightened approach, the way the hormonal differences between the sexes affects the way they interpret and respond to one another and the world around them. He reveals why women need a good supply of oxytocin and men, testosterone. He explains the impact of stress on hormonal balance, and how the stress of our modern lives is having far reaching effects on our relationships and our health.

One of John's true gifts is his ability to capture the essential nature of our differences and to explain them in terms that we can understand, providing practical tips and advice that anyone can follow. And you don't need a PhD, or to completely rebuild your life. Although there will always be some people who require greater care or personal counseling, John's approach allows most people to make improvements in their lives and loves simply and easily.

We not only can't separate the mind from the body, but we can't change one without changing the other. Our perspectives on life can have a huge impact on our emotional and physical health. Sometimes a slight shift in thinking can make a huge difference—between being sad or happy, between feeling anger or sympathy, or between giving up on our relationships or being able to flourish in them.

In *Venus on Fire Mars on Ice*, John shares the essential elements of wellness, happiness and lasting passion, revealing the keys to natural health and joyous vitality.

ABOUT HYLA CASS, M.D.

Hyla Cass, M.D., is a board certified psychiatrist, and internationally acclaimed innovator in the field of integrative medicine, emphasizing natural approaches to psychiatry, women's health, and hormonal issues. A frequent expert on national radio, television, and in national print media, she is also author of several popular books including *Natural Highs, 8 Weeks to Vibrant Health,* and *Supplement Your Prescription.*

CONTENTS

INTRODUCTION

MARS AND VENUS
IN A SHIFTING UNIVERSE

When I wrote *Men Are from Mars, Women Are from Venus* in 1992, my goal was to guide men and women to an understanding of their basic differences. The genders come from worlds practically next door to one another, yet in many ways, they may as well have come from opposite ends of the solar system. No wonder, I said, that the Venusians had trouble getting along with the Martians and vice-versa! Men from Mars are all about solutions, while women from Venus are about feelings. Women want to be loved, while men want to be needed. And both men and women tend to love the way they themselves want to be loved—not how their partner needs to be loved.

In that book and others that followed, I taught couples how to accept their differences, to work with them and to celebrate them. But never once did I say, "and this is *why* we are different." I couldn't. I didn't have the knowledge back then; nobody did.

Today we know! Some recent and very exciting scientific discoveries have proven that the difference between the sexes and how they relate to one another is biochemically based and can be found in... *our hormones*. These hormonal differences don't just determine whether we like to shop or fix things; they reveal the unique ways that each gender deals with stress. Without an adequate supply of these hormones onboard, our bodies suffer both mental and physical illness. But, with a plan in place to ensure ample production of these hormones, we find we have the strength and energy to cope with the challenges of our days. In other words, these break-through discoveries teach us things that are incredibly important for thriving in the fast-paced world we inhabit. *They tell us how to live, love, and achieve healthy longevity together.*

This new information couldn't come at a better time. A majority of today's women are working all day, only to come home and pull another shift on domestic duties. Men are struggling to hold jobs that are rapidly changing if not disappearing. Statistics show that men and women alike are sleeping less, eating worse and getting sicker. Divorce statistics remain high, and the number of women who stay single has increased by 100 percent. It's just plain hard to live in today's world. And it can be even harder to live in that world together, as a couple. And while life is getting harder, I'm happy to introduce simple and practical ways to enhance your relationships. Sometimes we complicate matters too much and simplicity can equal brilliance in your important relationships.

In this book I will give you the knowledge and simple tips required to ensure a steady supply of feel-good hormones for you and your partner's specific needs. I will teach you about stress hormones—specifically, the ways that they harm our health and complicate our ability to relate to one another. Along the way we'll talk about how good nutrition, balanced blood sugar, sound sleep and the addition of some exciting new dietary supplements that will aid you in replenishing the hormones you use up in the course of a stressful day. And, by applying your new hormonal knowledge to your daily interactions with your partner, you will find that the things that never quite made sense in your relationship now do!

So, join me in taking a light-hearted look at the fun and foibles of Mars and Venus as they learn to cope with a fast-evolving universe. Meet me inside to learn how you and your partner can use our newfound understanding of how men and women deal with stress to ensure a long life filled with love, happiness, and vitality.

You won't need to knock your world off its axis to achieve all this and more. All it takes is a few subtle shifts and simple changes—and a determination to see your most important relationship become more mutually supportive and fulfilling than you ever dreamed it could be.

CHAPTER 1

VENUS ON FIRE, MARS ON ICE—WHY?

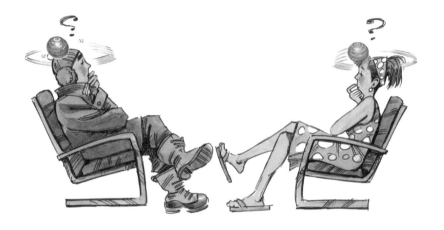

SHE WONDERS: WHY IS HE SO COLD?
HE WONDERS: WHY IS SHE SO ANGRY WITH ME?

He comes home after an exhausting day, looking forward to putting his feet up and relaxing in his favorite chair. He's ready to chill, read the news or watch TV. Finally, after a day of tackling problems on the job, he can just put the day's frustrations behind him. The last thing he wants is to deal with another problem. He's ready for a break. He wants a chance to cool down and forget his responsibilities.

She wonders, what's wrong? Is he ignoring me? Shouldn't he tell me about his day, or ask me about mine? Can't he do a few chores before he plops into a chair? Does he even see me here? In her mind, the concerns escalate. Why doesn't he want to talk to me? Why doesn't he participate in family life when he gets home? Why can't he open up and share his feelings? Is he taking me for granted? What happened to the man I married? Does he even love me anymore?

She wonders: Why is he so cold? (*Mars on Ice.*)

He wonders: Why is she so angry with me? (*Venus on Fire.*)

Sound familiar? Well, if men are from Mars and women are from Venus, then, at the end of the day or after a few years of marriage, quite often Venus is on Fire and Mars is on Ice. And until quite recently, we haven't had the scientific knowledge to understand why.

The Hormones of Fire and Ice

These opposing attributes—fire in women and ice in men—really do exist. Women and men aren't different because they grew up differently or came to look at the world in differing ways, though both can be true. It's because the bodies of men and women are hormonally poles apart. The biochemical makeup of the two genders is not the same. We have known this, in broad terms, for a long time. But it's only recently that we've gained the scientific knowledge to pinpoint which hormones are most influential in the success and failure of relationships. Understanding our gender-related hormonal differences provides us a revolutionary new perspective not only on improving our day-to-day efforts to relate to one another, but on how to create a lifetime's worth of health and happiness together.

Recent research has revealed that women release a hormone called oxytocin to cope with stress while men release testosterone for the same purpose. Oxytocin is released in safe, cooperative, caring, supportive and nurturing situations. Testosterone is something of an emergency hormone, released in situations that require urgency, sacrifice for a noble cause and problem solving. This hormonal difference offers us a keener understanding of why men and women so often fail to "get" one another. It's because men and women have very different biochemical needs when they seek to cope with stress—whether that's the big stress of a major loss or setback or the little stress of working through a to-do list.

	For Testosterone Release	For Oxytocin Release
1	Urgency and Emergency	Safe and Cooperative
2	Sacrifice for a Noble Cause	Caring and Supportive
3	Problem Solving	Nurturing Activities

This is a ground-breaking discovery for the newly emerging science of gender intelligence. It deserves our attention because it points both men and women in the right direction when seeking to handle the ups and downs of daily life. More importantly, it helps each side make sense of the opposite sex and the very different ways in which the other gender copes.

So for clarity, let's delve deeper into this remarkable hormonal discovery. Understanding the differing effects of oxytocin and testosterone on men and women is the first step in making the subtle shifts in behavior and nutrition we'll discuss in the rest of the book.

> For a man, increased levels of testosterone reduce stress. For a woman, increased levels of oxytocin reduce stress.

Let's start with men. When a man's hormonal testosterone level goes up, his stress level comes down. That's not true for a woman. Testosterone feels good to her because it gives her a sense of power and capability and makes her feel sexy, but it doesn't lower her stress level. Too much testosterone can cause aggression and impulsivity and, yes, it can actually raise a woman's level of stress.

To cope effectively with stress, a man is drawn to situations that either release testosterone or rebuild testosterone. Problem solving releases testosterone, which is why men enjoy fixing the toaster or changing the oil. As he acts, a man feels competent and powerful. But soon thereafter he needs to kick back and recover, because resting or taking time for recreation gives him a chance to rebuild his stores of testosterone. Take away either half of the cycle and I'll show you a man who is stressed out and probably not functioning very well.

Now let's look at women. When oxytocin levels go up in a woman, her stress levels come down. This is not true for a man.

The cycle of action and rest helps men cope effectively with stress.

Oxytocin feels good to him, increasing his tendencies toward trust, empathy, and generosity, but it's like testosterone in a woman—oxytocin doesn't lower his stress level. It may even increase it. Practically speaking, too much oxytocin can make a man sleepy and knock his testosterone level down significantly.

To cope effectively with stress, women are drawn to situations that stimulate the release of oxytocin and facilitate the rebuilding of oxytocin. By sharing herself in nurturing situations, oxytocin is released and her stress levels decline. By receiving nurturing sup-

The cycle of giving and receiving nurturing support helps women cope effectively with stress.

port, she is able to rebuild her oxytocin levels. This cycle of nurturing, then receiving nurturing support, then nurturing again, governs the life of a woman who is successful in coping with her stress. Deprive her of any part of it and she'll soon be feeling like she's stretched too thin.

When we talk about these stress-relieving hormones, it's important to remember that both genders make use of testosterone and oxytocin and derive benefit from each of these biochemical substances. But men and women differ greatly on how much of each hormone they need and how effectively they make it and store it.

Take testosterone. While it's a beneficial hormone for women, it's much more important for men. Without it, a man's stress level rises quickly. Think of the poor guy who goes to the mall with his wife. There's no problem for him to solve when she's shopping. There's no goal, either—as far as he can tell, she's going to shop forever! Without a problem to solve or a goal to meet, he's exhausted and frustrated and soon downright demoralized. He's not making any testosterone and must make a lot of it and fast, for he needs not 10 times more than a woman, but fully 30 times more. That, ladies, is why he seems magnetically pulled to the closest chair and it's also why it's such a struggle to get him out of that chair. Your man is in testosterone deficit, big-time! He needs far more of it than you.

Now let's look at oxytocin. Oxytocin is certainly beneficial to men, but it's much more important to women. It's not an issue of quantity, because women and men actually have similar levels of oxytocin. It's that women deplete their supply of oxytocin faster than men, and that's especially true when a woman is under stress. Availing themselves of opportunities to rebuild oxytocin levels by receiving nurturing support is the greatest unmet challenge for women today. Finding time to receive nurturing is often the last thing a woman is willing to do when she's under stress. She does more and more and more because, until now, she hasn't understood the role oxytocin plays in her well-being. With a new grasp on the hormonal dynamics in her life, any woman should be able to shift from always giving to taking the time she needs to receive support.

> Men must make 30 times more testosterone than women to recover from stress.

Balancing Work and Home Life

Back when men brought home the bacon and women stayed home to raise the children, things were more clear-cut, hormonally speaking. In the so-called ideal household of an earlier era, men knew they could relax when they came home in the evening. Because women had plenty of time to create a nurturing home they had very few expectations of a husband besides being a gentleman and a good provider. In this traditional arrangement, each gender had a better chance of having their hormonal storehouses replenished than we see today.

Today, balancing work and home life, business and personal life, has become a great challenge for most women and the men who love them. Each day a woman returns from one full-time job outside the home to another—inside the home. Whether she loves the job or simply needs it for economic reasons, working leaves her little or no time to relax and cope with stress. As she returns home from work and approaches the door, she's almost afraid to open it! That's because, inside, she faces a whole new set of responsibilities with nowhere near enough time to "do it all."

With more women in the workplace the stress at home has increased.

For many women, balancing work with the continued challenges of life at home is a goal that remains frustratingly out of reach. Making money and contributing to the family is great, many tell me, "but I'd kill for a good night's sleep!" And a romantic date with their husband. And a little help with the dishes. For too many women I know today, life is out of balance and relentlessly stressful.

Objective research backs up my anecdotal evidence. Cortisol is a major stress hormone, and studies measuring men's and women's cortisol levels reveal that women's stress levels at work are double those of a man. When she returns home, those stress levels increase even more. Meanwhile, a man who comes home to sit in his easy chair and watch the news sees his cortisol levels, which are already lower than hers, drop yet lower. His world didn't change much when women increased their representation in the workforce. But her world is off its axis. And that fact has led to what is perhaps the most significant difference between men of today, as opposed to men of, say, 1960. Today's husband has a wife with a list of complaints and needs that his father couldn't have imagined.

It used to be that women were measurably happier than men, but not anymore. While men have shown little change in happiness over the past 20 years, the average woman's happiness level as measured on psychological surveys has sunk like a stone. As a man who has been married for almost 25 years, I know that women's unhappiness is going to begin negatively affecting men's happiness levels and soon. There's a common saying, "When Mama ain't happy, ain't nobody happy." In my experience, it's true. When women suffer we all suffer.

When stress levels are moderate and well managed, both men and women can be at their best. They are warm and friendly as well as giving and appreciative to each other. But as stress increases, they

Women now score lower than men on tests that measure happiness.

change—and the change expresses itself in significantly different ways. Women feel overwhelmed with too much to do, while men either retreat to preoccupations with work or fall asleep on the couch. When home life no longer offers remedies for the stress of work, women tend to heat up while men become cold as ice.

Making Sense of our Differences

Here's where I think our improved understanding of hormonal influences makes a major contribution. Learning about testosterone and oxytocin and the differing effects they have on the two genders offers great hope for finding peace and mutual satisfaction in our relationships. Incorporating our new knowledge is crucial: Unless those of us in relationships understand our differing needs when we react to the stressors in our lives, we will experience ever-increasing tension and disillusionment. That's because failing to understand our partners at this basic, biochemical level allows unnecessary frustration, disappointment and concern to grow. Better we should gain a clear and specific understanding of the roles of testosterone and oxytocin and how they can help us make sense of one another. Let's explore a few common questions with new answers:

1. Question: Women commonly ask, *"How can he just sit there and watch TV when the house is a mess?"*

Answer: A man seeks out the couch or an easy chair after a stressful day because relaxing his muscles and putting the problems and responsibilities of the day out of his mind rebuilds his testosterone levels. He may not notice the mess, or if he does, it doesn't bother him. He's got higher priorities.

2. Question: Men commonly ask, *"Why does she always want to talk about her day? Even worse, why does she want me to talk about my day?"*

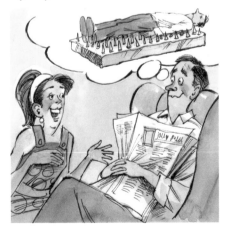

Answer: A woman seeks out nurturing activities as a way of rebuilding her oxytocin levels and reducing her stress. That's why she wants her man to talk about his day. When a man listens supportively as she describes her day, this also helps rebuild her oxytocin levels.

3. Question: Women commonly ask, *"What's the big deal with watching TV? Why is he more interested in TV than in me? And furthermore, why does he insist on having a big-screen TV?"*

> **Answer:** Studies have shown that when a man is relaxing and watching TV his testosterone levels are rebuilding and increasing, reducing his stress. As to the second part of the question, I'd say that size does matter. Little TV, little testosterone. Big TV—well, you get the picture!

4. Question: Men commonly ask, *"Why does she get so upset about things? Why can't she just chill? Most of what she talks about doesn't seem like such a big deal to me, so why is it so important to her to talk about it?"*

> **Answer:** It's a big deal to her. Under moderate stress, women have a much bigger reaction in the emotional part of the brain. Talking about her feelings helps her to feel seen, heard, understood and loved. This, in turn, rebuilds and releases her anti-stress hormone, oxytocin.

5. Question: Women commonly ask, *"Why does he always wait until the last minute to do things? He waits to pack for trips, he waits to plan our dates, he waits to buy presents, and he never washes dishes until they're piled sky high."*

> **Answer:** When a man puts off doing things, it's because it's in his nature to let the pressure build up until it would be dangerous to wait any longer. Remember, it's his sense of risk, danger and the need for problem solving that stimulate the release of testosterone. This, in turn, lowers his stress and gives him the extra energy boost or motivation to get the job done.

6. Question: Men commonly ask, *"Why is she always planning things? I think she worries too much. Why can't she just relax and not take on so much?"*

Answer: When a woman cares about others and shows it by planning events for them, it's a nurturing act that releases oxytocin. While a man carries a wallet and a comb, just the essentials, a woman carries a big purse with everything she or anyone else (family, friends, co-workers) could possibly need. On Venus, planning ahead is an act of caring and consideration that releases oxytocin to help her cope with stress.

7. Question: Women commonly ask, *"Where did all the romance go? In the beginning he would plan dates, give me compliments and show me lots of affection. Now he only touches me when he wants sex."*

Answer: In the beginning of your relationship, he was solving a problem: getting you to love him! As he worked on it, that "problem" released his testosterone, lowered his stress and gave him plenty of romantic energy. Now that you're married, there's a new set of problems to solve, like paying the mortgage. Romance doesn't release his stress-busting testosterone anymore, but being seen as a good provider does.

8. Question: Men commonly ask, *"Why do I have to jump through hoops to have a sex life? She complains that I'm not affectionate enough and that there's not enough romance or intimacy."*

Answer: Women love sex just as much as men do. It's oxytocin that sometimes makes it seem like you have to fill out paperwork and be officially pre-qualified for intimacy with her. If her oxytocin level is low, her sex drive is diminished and her stress level is high. If her oxytocin level is high, perhaps due to the stress-reducing effect of your care and attention, her sexual response may be very strong indeed. Kind words and considerate actions count for a lot! Later on, we'll explore easy and practical ways for men to stimulate high levels of oxytocin in the women they love. As you'll see, it's a new approach that, with her help, can do wonders to invigorate your love life.

Here we can see that, as the result of our new understanding of the stress-reducing effects of hormones, all the old questions women and men have asked about one another for generations now have new answers. Answers that explain rather than excuse. Answers that help us make sense of a situation instead of throwing up our hands in desperation. This information isn't found in most relationship books because most of it was, until recently, unknown or unproven.

Our opportunity to gain greater mutual understanding in our relationship is unprecedented. Think of it: We won't jump to (wrong) conclusions when we have a newly-achieved grasp of what's really going on. We won't blame our partners when things go wrong, because we know that most conflicts are rooted in the basic, biochemical differences between us—things that get "fixed" when they are understood. Instead of feeling confused or powerless, we can begin to formulate a whole new way to interact and relate. This is exciting stuff! Now that we know why Venus is on fire and Mars is on ice, we can focus our efforts on ensuring that our partner, whom we love above all else, gets what he or she needs—while never sacrificing what we ourselves want and need. Finding this balance begins with making sense of one another in a new and positive way.

Colliding Together In Love

In far too many once-great relationships, the man quits trying to meet his partner's needs and grows distant. At the same time, the woman may become dissatisfied with her man's lack of understanding and stop giving him her trust. He becomes more passive. She becomes more demanding. No matter how hard they try, the pair can't seem to reclaim the easy and generous atmosphere of love and happiness they enjoyed when they first came together.

It would be nice if I could tell you that understanding the distinction between fire and ice is the answer in such a situation.

Mars and Venus can collide—yet still grow in deeper love and compassion.

Unfortunately, I can't, because the sad truth is that information alone is not enough. It takes knowledge plus a positive attitude. Seen negatively, differences between men and women can become the force that pushes planets apart. But when Venus and Mars can see their differences appreciatively, the two planets become capable of closer, more harmonious orbit.

There will be collisions; there always are. But, instead of seeing these planetary bumps as blights on our relationship, we can come to view these events as opportunities to learn more about each other and forgive one another. In so doing, we grow closer together instead of further apart. Recognizing and remembering that we are supposed to be different helps to soften our hearts so that we can come together in love. Thus, a relationship become perfect for us as we learn, day by day, to love and accept each other's natural tendencies as something other than imperfections.

Understanding how and why our partners respond as they do can help improve any relationship, no matter the age or stage. Knowing the ways that men and women cope with stress on a physical, hormonal level frees us from feeling hopeless, or worse, feeling wounded by our partner's actions and reactions.

As our mutual insight grows, we begin to recognize that we have a choice as to whether we bring out the best in our partners or the worst. We discover that increasing our understanding of one another opens our hearts and releases us from our tendency to judge others.

Too often we make assumptions about our partner that intensify our feelings of discontent and prevent us from expressing the love that lives in our hearts. The following story, shared with me by a friend, illustrates the transformational power of gaining new understanding and perspective. I will share this story as it was told to me.

"One day I came home and discovered a car parked next to my driveway, in my favorite parking spot. My first reaction was annoyance, because even though it was street parking, I felt I owned that spot. I always parked there! Now I had to park farther away, and carry my stuff farther, too. For several hours I obsessed about who was in my spot, grumbling to my wife about how inconsiderate he was and checking repeatedly to see if the car was still there. Eventually I even went outside to have a closer look.

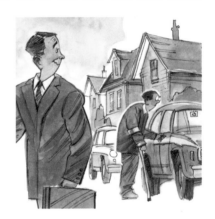

"Suddenly a man came out of the house across the street and started to walk towards the offending car. It was immediately obvious to me that he had a physical handicap that made walking difficult and, in all probability, painful. As I was taking this in, he looked at me, smiled and said hello. In that moment of understanding, all my previous annoyance completely evaporated and I found myself filled with compassion and concern. I didn't care anymore that he was in 'my' spot—instead I imagined how glad he must have been to be able to park close to his destination. How challenging his life must be compared to mine, I thought. I wanted to find out more about him, to get to know him, maybe even to help in some bigger way.

"I realized then how easily I had fallen into the trap of jumping to a negative conclusion instead of imagining that there could be a good reason for that car to be there. Instead of putting myself in someone else's shoes and responding with openness and a positive attitude, I got angry. We are all damaged in one way or another, even if it's not visible on the surface. We should remember to be kind, patient and understanding of others, because we don't know what burdens they may be carrying."

I love this story because it illustrates how quickly our judgments, resentments and tendencies toward rejection can disappear when we understand a situation differently; when we can imagine what it is like to walk the world in another's shoes. I hope that when your partners are parking where you don't want them to, you can use your newfound knowledge to see the world through their eyes and their hormones, and that you, too, can experience an epiphany that leads to greater compassion and love. I hope each of you will use this book to gather the facts you need to release the past, open your heart, and give yourself and your partner another chance—not once or twice, but again and again.

In Chapter Two we'll explore how stress hormones such as cortisol affect our health, sometimes for good but mostly for ill. We'll also see how the anti-stress hormones, testosterone, and oxytocin, are creating a revolution in hormonal health for those who pay heed to the research. As you will read, more and more doctors, health researchers, teachers and others are pointing the way to increased happiness and better health by increasing your body's access to beneficial hormones and stress-reducing brain chemicals. All of this is yours for the taking, simply by making subtle changes in how you nourish your body and relate to the people who mean the most to you. You can experience a positive impact on your life and your relationship—simply by reading on.

CHAPTER 2

VENUS AND MARS UNDER STRESS

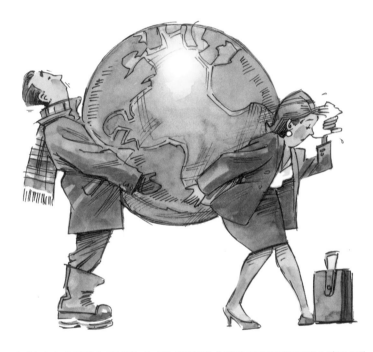

BOTH MEN AND WOMEN ARE EXPERIENCING
STRESS AT UNPRECEDENTED LEVELS.

There is no such thing as a bad hormone. Your teenage self might have disagreed on that point, but it's true: Each hormonal substance our body makes has something positive and useful about it, as long as we have it available to us at the right time and in the right amount.

Balance is key. Get too little of a particular hormone and you have one set of problems or issues. Get too much, and the list of negative effects is just as long, though different. Still, if I had to name one hormone that is causing harm in modern daily life, it would be cortisol, the stress hormone.

Our ancestors would strongly disagree. After all, they would say, wasn't it cortisol that helped their next-cave neighbor outrun that bear? Didn't cortisol give their auntie the strength to pull a drowning child out of a raging river?

It's true. Cortisol is a lifesaver. It's what gives firefighters the courage to run fearlessly into a burning building and get out again safely. It's what gets a backpacker over the mountain in record time as lightning flashes in the sky. It's also what helps us cope with a crucial job interview, a merciless deadline or the emergency surgery of a loved one. When cortisol levels rise, our body is able to react quickly to peril. When the danger passes—the bear lumbers away, the storm ends, the surgery is successful—cortisol levels fall. The exertion of dealing with the stressor uses up the cortisol that the body's adrenal gland produced.

At least that's how it's supposed to work. Our bodies are designed to experience brief bursts of stress-induced cortisol release. As danger passes and relaxation occurs, cortisol levels should fall. Elevated cortisol levels are not meant to stay elevated.

And that's why I say cortisol is the closest thing we have to a bad hormone. Indeed, when cortisol stays in our systems for too long, it has poisonous effects. Cortisol ages us prematurely, plays with our emotions and is linked to many a life-threatening disease.

Clearly, it's in our best interests to manage our cortisol production. And the good news is that we can. In this chapter we will consider some very powerful ways of keeping the stress hormone, cortisol, from stressing us out. Yes, there are things we can do to protect our bodies and our relationships from the negative effects of this powerful substance.

Stress and the Hormone Cortisol

Let's back up a moment to consider what stress actually is. Generally speaking, when we use the word stress we're referring to circumstances outside ourselves that we don't like or over which we have little control. These days it's likely to mean heavy traffic, unreturned phone calls, overdue bills or missed travel connections. Add to the list interpersonal matters such as finding a date for Saturday night, broaching a difficult subject with a spouse, or asking a boss for a raise, and you soon see that assessing stress is quite individual and very subjective. But there is an objective measurement of stress in the body: *Your cortisol level.*

In response to stressors, our adrenal glands release the hormone cortisol in the amount the situation seems to require. When our response to stressors is moderate, cortisol levels rise modestly. When our response to stressors is great, cortisol levels rise sharply. We may feel the overproduction of cortisol in the form of anxiety or tension, but then again, we may not feel anything at all. Yet, when our cortisol level is chronically elevated, damage is occurring.

There are several other facts to keep in mind about stress. First, different people experience it differently. What winds you up way too tightly might barely cause a reaction in someone else. Second, stress can't be made to go away. It's a part of life. So our mission, if we are to live happy, healthy lives, is not to try to make stress go away, because it won't. Nor is it to hope that someone invents a home cortisol test to

> Managing stress effectively is more about changing our reaction to stress than attempting to avoid stressful situations.

tell us when our stress hormones are getting too high, or a cortisol antidote to take to neutralize it. No, the mission is to change our reaction to stress.

This is easier said than done. The dice is loaded and the deck is stacked against us. Just think for a moment about our lives. We are sedentary. Many of us confront our stresses at a desk, in a workplace where we suffer from limited control over the things that worry us. Procrastinating may be seen as a way of running away from our problems, but the opportunity to really run away has been lost to the ages. Our office-bound bodies are steeped in cortisol that we aren't getting rid of. And the stressors just keep coming.

This would be fine if the adrenal gland had an off switch. But the adrenal gland only sees the peril and the need to produce cortisol to respond to it. Nothing tells the gland, "It's okay, go ahead and stop; we've already got more than we need." The result? An overworked adrenal gland that over-produces cortisol and under-produces the stress-fighting hormones that each gender needs—testosterone for men and oxytocin for women.

Let me state this in a different way: The way we live today, with our many stresses big and small, the body's adrenal gland is working extra shifts. The continual and ever-increasing demand for cortisol has two unfortunate consequences. The adrenal gland gets worn out and can't produce cortisol as effectively. More importantly, the body's continual demand for cortisol means that this little hormone factory almost abandons its other product lines. We'll get to that in a moment, but first...

Let's review: When we're stressed out while sitting at our desks or while driving our cars, three things can happen:

1	Cortisol is released and we don't use it up by physically running away from danger.
2	Cortisol is released and it remains high because we continue facing or thinking about problems we can't immediately escape from.
3	Eventually less cortisol is released because the adrenal gland is exhausted.

These three responses produce a variety of unintended, undesirable and unhealthy consequences. They trigger a cascade of reactions that is responsible for nearly every health challenge we experience today.

Starved for Hormones?

With the chart above, we've now laid the groundwork to fully understand something that sounds impossible but isn't: Both men and women today are actually running out of hormones. Few of us are getting the hormones we need, when we need them. And it's because they aren't there to be gotten! The shelves are empty. The bottom of the barrel has been scraped. Is it an issue of aging? No, getting older doesn't cause low levels of hormones, although low hormone levels do cause us to age prematurely.

The primary cause of hormone deficiency is sustained high levels of cortisol. Cortisol is the culprit that shuts down the production of the other hormones our bodies need. Why? Well, for all the millions of people who have pondered the question, science has now provided us the answer, right here in the next sentence: When the adrenal gland is releasing cortisol, your body stops making the other health-producing hormones, two of which are the stress reducers, testosterone for men and oxytocin for women.

> Under stress, the body stops making the feel-good hormones that keep us healthy and happy.

This is why it's so crucial to find ways of reducing stress. Stress stimulates cortisol production and overtaxes the adrenal glands. By lowering cortisol levels and supporting the adrenal gland, the body returns to producing an abundance of all the right hormones. It's really as simple as that.

Over the past 10 years, equipped with this new understanding, I have personally helped thousands of individuals restore healthy hormone production, sometimes within weeks or even days. We'll delve into this further, right after we figure out why Mother Nature would create a biochemical system that allows us to live with hormonal deficit.

Why the Hormonal Well Runs Dry

Survival, that's why. Underlying the whys and wherefores of our biological processes is one powerful drive: continuation of the species. Under normal conditions, the body makes an abundant supply of the most important survival hormones like testosterone so that men are interested in sex. Testosterone gives a man the energy and motivation to do what it takes to find and impress a mate with whom he can procreate. In women, the baby-making is made possible by an abundance of progesterone and estrogen. All three of the hormones I just mentioned, along with others, are derived from what is known as the mother hormone, DHEA. Without DHEA, the survival of the species is over.

It's business as usual for the body to produce these biochemical substances. As long as you're providing your body the right nutritional support, it's really no feat at all to make an abundance of life-giving, species-preserving—and stress-reducing—hormones. No hormone supplements or replacements are needed. However, when the adrenal gland is making cortisol, the gland recognizes it as a lifesaver and gives it the highest priority. It's like a factory pressed into wartime service. All normal production comes to a stop. All assembly lines previously devoted to testosterone, oxytocin, estrogen, progesterone and others are shut down. The body retains its ancient knowledge and performs a time-tested threat assessment. The conclusion? "If I don't get away from this bear, I won't need to worry about feeling good or making babies ever again."

> To improve our health and relationships, we need to fix the broken switch on the adrenal gland's assembly line.

To ensure survival, the adrenal gland shifts from making DHEA to making cortisol. Once we've escaped from danger and run off the cortisol we produced, the body relaxes and goes back to business as usual, creating an abundance of hormones. Of course, as we've already discussed, too many of us today have cortisol production facilities that operate just about full-time. The switch is stuck "on."

Clearly, what we must do is to fix the switch so that we produce only the cortisol we need, when we need it. This will allow our beleaguered adrenal gland to get back to making the stress-reducing hormones we've been running out of. It will also preserve or restore our own health and improve the quality of our relationships.

You might think that fixing the switch requires a biochemical solution of some kind, and that's partly true. In chapters to come, you will learn more about foods and supplements that can become part of your toolbox as you seek to live the happiest, healthiest, most loving life you can.

But you need to feed your mind as much—or even more—than your body! You'll achieve better and faster results if you focus on tuning up your relationship with the opposite sex, that Martian or Venusian who shares your household. In my consulting practice I've found that both men and women benefit when they take the time to gain a thorough understanding of how each gender copes with stress. We touched on this topic in Chapter One, and introduced you to the concept of improved relationships through hormone-based stress reduction. Now it's time to expand on that information.

Picture a couple, a man and a woman, who have been together for a few years or more, both of whom have significant levels of responsibility in their daytime lives. Each knows the other is busy. Still, at home in the evening, there's a strong tendency for both the man and the woman to underestimate one another's stress levels.

Objectively, we know this is crazy. Due to our fast-paced lives, both men and women are experiencing stress at unprecedented levels. With time- and labor-saving devices everywhere we look, logic tells us we should be less stressed, but the opposite is true.

When I talk about the enormous stress that women are experiencing today, some husbands living in America naively reply, "My wife isn't stressed; she's better off than 99 percent of the world's population!" This is a man who doesn't understand what stress really is. Basically, he's saying, "What does she have to complain about? We have a house and plenty of food in the refrigerator."

This attitude is just plain ignorant, and it can destroy a relationship. What such a man doesn't know or isn't accepting is that there are different kinds of stress. Poverty and the threat of starvation is one kind of stress. Living in a country with few opportunities for economic advancement is a different kind of stress. We are indeed lucky that most of us don't live under such circumstances. But, believe it or not, these kinds of stress are actually very low compared to the kinds of stress men and women are experiencing in the modern world. Living life in a hurry while stuck in L.A. traffic can produce much higher levels of stress, as measured by cortisol levels, than living in a rural village with no electricity, no grocery stores, and little opportunity to live a better life.

So, it's clear that at least some men misunderstand and underestimate their partner's stress.

Let's look at what's really going on with women: Almost 40 percent of women in America today are their family's primary breadwinner. Soon, the majority of workers in the U.S. may be women. That's unprecedented, and so is the amount of wealth that women control. What generations of women strove to accomplish—gaining more access to money and opportunity—seems to have been achieved. Yet, women face harder choices, greater unhappiness and, yes, higher levels of stress than ever. Why?

> Hurried lives create enormous stress even when our physical needs are being met.

Survey after survey shows that though women want greater responsibility in the workplace and are achieving it, their anxiety about financial security has grown to levels greater than their male counterparts. That's one thing. It's also true that women would feel more fulfilled and make more of the stress-reducing hormone, oxytocin, if they would recognize their need to nurture. But these days that's not always possible. With mom filling ever more important roles in the workplace, stay-at-home dads are found in up to 11 percent of married couples.

Let's not leave homemakers out of the discussion. These women, too, are experiencing very high levels of stress. Shopping, cooking, cleaning and raising children is the sort of nurturing activity that raises the production of oxytocin, the hormone that reduces stress for women. But it's work that can be draining and stress-producing if a woman feels unappreciated and unsupported. If she's managing the household in a vacuum (as well as with one!), traditional homemaking activities can become another source of stress. It can be an isolating existence, especially if the woman can't find the support of a network of other mothers. Where are the other mothers? Working outside the home, most likely. My conclusion is that, whether a woman's work is full-time outside the home or as a stay-at-home mother, her personal life is too often not the source of support she would like it to be. Men may not be the problem, but they're not often the solution, either. I won't just pick on men.

Women are also guilty of underestimating their partner's stress, but mostly because she thinks he's got ample opportunity to loaf. She looks at him there on the couch and thinks, "It sure must be nice to just flop at the end of the day." She has a point, because it's true that she's moving around a lot more than he is. She thinks, "Why is he lying leisurely on the couch instead of helping me?" She probably has no idea that sitting or lying down on a couch is one of the best ways for a man to make testosterone and recover from stress. Without this insight, she'll think or say, "Why does he get to lie down?" As if lying down was even an option for her!

Actually, each partner is doing what he or she ought to do. As much as men and women need to recognize their partner's high stress level, they also need to appreciate the differing ways they each cope with it.

Relaxing on a couch reduces stress for men. Getting nurturing support reduces stress for women.

Normally, unless a woman is totally exhausted, lying down has little value to her in reducing stress. For her, resting on the couch only provides a minimal amount of relief. She'd soon feel restless, thinking of all the things she needs to get done. Moving around and working on her to-do list feels better. Men aren't doing their wives any favors by getting irritated and saying, "Can't you just sit still for one minute and relax?" Sitting on the couch or doing some enjoyable activity independently is one of the best ways for men to recover from stress, but that's just not true for women.

As we've already explored, a man copes best with stress by alternatingly taking action to solve problems with time for rest and recreation. A woman, on the other hand, needs to balance giving to others with taking time to give herself support or receive support from others. Resting rebuilds testosterone, the anti-stress hormone for men, while receiving nurturing support rebuilds oxytocin, the anti-stress hormone for women.

What must men and women do so they both feel happy, healthy and fulfilled in the roles they now play? They must recognize that love and stress reduction are virtually one and the same, coming as they do from the same hormonal source.

Hormones of Love, Desire, and Longevity

You have come to know oxytocin and testosterone as stress-reducers, but they have a romantic side as well. Oxytocin is the hormone of love, while testosterone is the hormone of desire. When women are feeling happy and in love, their oxytocin levels are high. When men are feeling motivated, passionate and romantic, their testosterone levels are high. These hormones of desire and love aren't just the foundation of lasting passion in our relationships, but of good health as well. That's because oxytocin and testosterone are scarce commodities in bodies flooded with stress-related cortisol.

We've already discussed from a biochemical perspective the problem of cortisol overproduction and the adrenal gland's associated tendency to quit producing oxytocin and testosterone. Now let's spend a little time looking at the same phenomenon from an interpersonal standpoint:

Low Oxytocin in Women: As a woman ages, and particularly after many years of marriage, the innocent exuberance of love and the generosity of an open heart are often lost to her. The young woman who delighted in just being taken out on a date complains later in life that her husband forgot to make reservations. She still loves him, but no longer feels in love. A part of her is held back now, remembering disappointments over the years. When the abundance of love in her heart is no longer easy to feel or share, her oxytocin levels are low.

> Oxytocin in women and testosterone in men enhance feelings of romance.

Low Testosterone in Men: Likewise, in a man, the natural motivation and desire to make a difference in romance becomes jaded through years of disappointment and frustration. The caring young man who eagerly planned ways to please his partner gradually resigns his fate to mediocre contentment. Rather than planning a date, he waits until Friday night to ask his wife what she'd like to do that night. While he thinks he's being loving, he doesn't have a clue that his actions indicate that the romance is gone. He's happy, but completely unaware of the passion and fulfillment that he has lost. When he forgets to plan dates and stops being interested in her day, it's not that he doesn't love her but that his testosterone levels are low.

Fully feeling love, passion, and desire is directly linked to an abundance of testosterone in men and oxytocin in women. For years I've focused on helping young couples keep these feelings alive—and helping older couples to rekindle them—by teaching men about women and women about men. With the help of science, I gained an understanding of the gender-specific anti-stress hormones that are the subject of this book. The new frontier, both for me and for others who explore the orbits of Mars and Venus, is the growing realization that the hormones of love, desire, and stress reduction are also the precursors to the hormones of health and longevity.

Relationships and Your Health

At first, the idea that changing the way you relate to others dramatically affects your health seems a stretch, maybe even ridiculous. Yet, more and more researchers are coming to this conclusion.

Many of the diseases that currently plague our society are now being called lifestyle diseases. This means that our stressful lifestyle directly causes heart disease, cancer, diabetes, and other killers. It's no longer a surprise that when people come to the U.S. their health deteriorates as they adopt the American lifestyle.

Studies have shown that Chinese immigrants, who are generally much healthier than Americans, began taking on the common diseases rampant in our society within a few years of arriving on our shores. At first this was considered to be the direct result of eating our less-healthy diet. However, a study was conducted of a particular group of Chinese immigrants that didn't adopt an American diet. They, too, were getting sicker! The researchers concluded that the primary cause of their increase in disease was their change in lifestyle and their separation from the cultural support they received in their home country.

Don't overlook the last few words of that previous sentence. Researchers at the prestigious Scripps Clinic in San Diego have concluded that heart disease is most often triggered by unresolved emotional issues like financial stress, divorce, loneliness or the inability to effectively communicate with a child or spouse. The connection may not be obvious, because it usually takes one or two years after the emotional trauma for the health problem to surface. But it's there.

This kind of research is often ignored or dismissed because people feel they have no power to change their lifestyles or reduce their stress. The good news is that we can change the way stress affects our bodies, even if we can't change the world. There's no magic wand to wave, but by understanding the gender-specific anti-stress hormones and how to maximize them in our lives, we can free ourselves from many of the negative effects of modern life. By making a few small changes in our lifestyle to improve the quality of our relationships, we can indeed make dramatic changes in our health.

Now, don't misunderstand what I've said. To look at the research that links our relationships to our health and conclude that the quality of our relationships determines who gets sick would be a big mistake. The point is more complex. It's not that our relationships make us sick. Rather, our lifestyle doesn't help our relationships stimulate the production of the right hormones to keep us healthy.

You could have very loving friends but not have time to share your friendship with them. You could love your family members very much but not get to see them very often. And, as is the case with many inhabitants of both Mars and Venus, you could have a great marriage, but come home too exhausted from work to create good communication or romance.

We can change the way stress affects our bodies, even if we can't change the world.

Our new understanding of the gender-specific hormones of love, desire, and stress-reduction helps us make the logical link between the quality of our relationships and our health. When you begin to make sense of how you can use your relationships to stimulate and produce these special anti-stress hormones of testosterone and oxytocin, the puzzle pieces practically fall into place.

Think of it: Anyone who has ever been in love knows that when you're sharing love, feeling loved or giving love, you feel wonderful. This feeling of "wonderful" is actually the release of stress, the dissipation of cortisol levels. It's the blissful return to the present moment where worries, concerns and fears have no power over our state of being. Unless we have an abundance of the right type of hormone, this state is rarely achieved. We now know if the anti-stress hormone levels are low, no matter how loving your partner is, you don't feel loved.

Recognizing that men and women cope differently with stress gives us a new tool for quickly and effectively lowering our stress levels, thus giving our exhausted adrenal gland a chance to recuperate. When we do that, we directly stimulate the production of health-producing hormones. Once we really understand the differing circumstances under which men and women produce these hormones, we can better support ourselves and our partners in coping with stress.

As we are seeing, a good relationship can become the foundation on which we build production and release of beneficial hormones. But more is required. It also takes a program encompassing diet, lifestyle, and exercise to provide the raw materials to make the anti-stress hormones. Without the right raw materials, even our relationships cannot keep us healthy and happy. In the next chapter we'll explore the new mind/body science that acknowledges hormones as the essential link for healthy longevity.

CHAPTER THREE

VENUS AND MARS OUT OF ORBIT

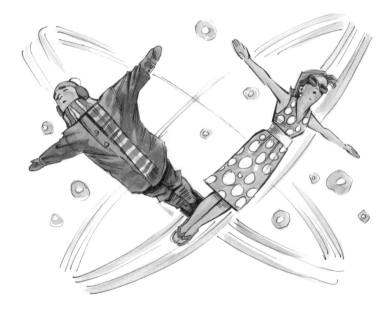

STRIVING TO BALANCE CHEMICALS HELPS MARS
AND VENUS STAY IN COMPATIBLE ORBITS.

The ancient Greeks understood that the mind and body are intimately connected: A healthy mind supports a healthy body; a healthy body supports a healthy mind. They didn't understand the exact nature of the connection. But today, thanks to abundant scientific research, we can take this insight to a whole new level.

New mind/body research shows us the missing link. It's to be found in our hormones. Our mind affects our hormones which then regulate our body. In turn, hormones powerfully affect what we think and feel. It's a complicated interaction that can't be overestimated and shouldn't be underappreciated. Indeed, even our moods have been shown to be directly related to our hormone levels and the balanced or unbalanced nature of our brain chemicals. A long time ago it was just a fantasy to think that there would be a "smile pill" capable of lifting a bad mood, or pills for sleeping or getting work done, but, as we all know, those pills have arrived in truckloads. Doctors can't write the prescriptions fast enough for all the depressed, weary or stressed patients coming their way.

The modern world's widespread dependence on antidepressants, sleeping pills, and amphetamines has become epidemic. An estimated one in five Americans has become dependent on some type of medication intended to help them cope effectively with life's stressors. In my consulting work, I learned of one hospital where half of the 20,000 employees were taking antidepressants. This is shocking.

New research reveals that hormones create an important link between the body and the mind.

I consider it a clear indictment of our way of life, especially since this dependence on prescription drugs is the direct consequence of our failure to support the health and well-being of our bodies.

When people talk about stress, they usually talk about factors related to their work or non-work commitments. But the stress of our busy lives is not merely due to our vocations and avocations. Whether we can sense it or not, our stress is increased and aggravated by our inability to recover from our outside-world stresses at home. When our personal relationships don't serve to lower our stress levels, our perception of stress and our symptoms of stress are bound to rise dramatically. That's when we reach for a pill—something to help us sleep, or get the work done, or simply to not feel so blue about it all.

More than twice as many women as men take antidepressants. There's good reason for today's women to try to address their mood disorders, because as we've already seen, modern women are experiencing (1) unprecedented levels of stress for their gender and (2) higher levels of stress than men. What accounts for the gender difference in antidepressant use? Brain differences.

One study has revealed that during a moderately stressful situation, a woman's brain has eight times more blood flow in the emotional part of the brain than a man's does in a similar situation. In fact, moderate stress hardly registers a reaction in a man's brain. But a woman's brain is strongly activated. Faced with something she regards as a threat, a woman draws upon her emotional memory. To anticipate possible danger, she remembers in clear detail many things that have gone wrong in similar situations in the past. Remember, this isn't just cognitive memory. It's emotional memory. She feels those past episodes and releases cortisol to meet the new challenge.

This explains why men commonly think women are "getting upset over nothing," and why women commonly think "men have no feelings." His brain only registers a strong emotional reaction when the problem is an emergency or at least has a sense of strong urgency. He's fully capable of experiencing the same level of emotional intensity that a woman does, but only when the situation is life-and-death dire. That's why everyday stressors that send Venus into orbit will have Mars wondering why she's overreacting.

But he's the one who's overreacting! He thinks she's declaring an emergency when she's not. Yes, she's upset. But she doesn't want or need to call 911. She wants only to share her feelings.

He says, "Why are you making such a big deal out of this?"

She says, "I'm not making a big deal out of it. I'm just telling you what happened."

He says, "If it's not a big deal, then why can't you just forget about it?"

She says, "I don't want to forget about it. I want to talk about it. Why can't you just listen?"

There it is, the battle of the sexes in a nutshell. On Mars, under moderate stress, you cope with stress by taking time to relax and put it out of your mind. If you can't do anything about it, the Martians figure, why not forget about it until you can do something? On Venus, they have a different custom, "If you can't do anything about a problem, you should at least talk about it."

Fine, but why is it that women are so determined to talk about their problems, even when the issue isn't urgent and they aren't really looking for a solution? Science now answers the question that people have been asking for centuries. When there is extra blood flow to the emotional part of the brain, a person begins to feel distressed. The brain's preferred response is to release a calming, feel-good brain chemical called serotonin, but it doesn't always happen as automatically as we might like. What women know intuitively is that talking about problems stimulates the release of serotonin. From the perspective of brain chemicals and stress hormones, then, it's clear that women talk about problems to calm the blood flow in the emotional part of their brain.

> Under moderate stress, women cope by talking, men cope by relaxing.

Normally, the human brain stores abundant serotonin, usually enough to handle occasional moments of stress. However, at the end of a grinding day, a woman can find herself fresh out of serotonin while the man still has plenty left. He doesn't need to talk to stimulate the release of more serotonin, but she craves the conversation. He doesn't understand her need to talk. That's because he has no idea how helpful talking and feeling heard can be for her. Meanwhile, she doesn't understand his lack of interest in the process. Doesn't he care?

Well, he certainly would care if he understood how much she needs the serotonin that talking can give her. When a woman feels emotionally supported by being able to share her feelings, it gives her the same sense of coping that a man might gain from "fixing" the situation. Talking rebuilds her serotonin supplies and calms her down. This, men, is why it's important sometimes to just listen and not try to solve her problems for her.

Our Brains Need a Steady Fuel Supply

But I have another factor to introduce to the equation: blood sugar. The body requires a steady supply of blood sugar to make serotonin. Indeed, no amount of talking will be sufficient to make serotonin and calm her brain if a woman has low blood sugar. With this scientific fact in hand, we can see that stabilizing blood sugar is at least as important as balancing hormones.

As you know, I've built a career on helping men and women learn to understand one another. I have emphasized the power of a loving relationship not just for the sake of harmony, but for health. Striving to balance chemicals such as testosterone, oxytocin, and serotonin has given me another tool to help Mars and Venus stay in compatible orbit. But, for me, the role of blood sugar has been an eye-opener. We now know that it's the lynchpin in terms of understanding the effect of brain chemistry on relationships. And, like so much we discuss in this book, we find that blood sugar is more important to women than it is to men.

If women are to benefit from the many stress-reducing benefits of a loving relationship, it's essential that they have a steady supply of fuel for their brains. The fuel is blood sugar. It can't be stored by the brain, and it must be kept within a narrow range of blood concentration to avoid stressing the brain. As the brain functions, it needs to draw steady supplies of energy in the form of sugar or glucose from the blood. Without ready access to blood sugar, a brain under stress can't make the serotonin it needs to relax and feel good again. Any time blood sugar surges too high or drops too low, brain chemistry is immediately thrown out of balance. As we've seen, the issue is most critical for women because they tend to deplete their supplies of serotonin more easily than do men. Remember, that's because more women are in the workplace making more testosterone and less of the stress-busting oxytocin they need, resulting in skyrocketing rates of cortisol, the stress hormone. No wonder women's brains go through serotonin as if it were ice cream.

This may seem like an odd place to insert a travel tip, but I've got a good one: Men, if you're traveling with your wife or girlfriend and she mentions that it's time to start looking for a restaurant, you need to sit up and take notice. This means her blood sugar level has dropped and, for you, it ought to be a red alert with flashing lights and sirens. Get that woman fed!

When a woman is hungry, it means her blood sugar levels have dropped to the point that she can't make serotonin until she refuels. This happens more readily to women than to men, because men generally have higher levels of blood sugar to begin with and don't have the dramatic fluctuations that women can experience over the course of a day.

A friendly tip for traveling couples: When the woman is hungry, feed her!

So, for the man seeking to have a nice day with the woman in his life, it's important to know that she can be feeling fine one minute and be thinking about food the next. Pay attention to the clues of depleted blood sugar. Your well-being depends on it! If she's hungry and stressed, you may easily find yourself in the proverbial doghouse for something you did hours, days or years ago. Nothing you can say will help. Take it from the man who's learned from experience: Just feed her fast, or she may experience selective amnesia and forget every good thing you've ever done in your life. Don't argue; it's like pouring gasoline on a fire. Just listen, nod, and... find her a restaurant!

Later in this chapter we'll talk more about the importance of maintaining a diet that supports a steady level of blood sugar. But first I want to give you a reason to really take that information to heart. Could it be true that many of the major symptoms of menopause are actually caused by highly-irregular blood sugar?

Is it Hormones or Blood Sugar?

It's true. New research reveals that the usual menopausal symptoms that run the gamut from weight gain to mood swings to hot flashes aren't necessarily caused by hormonal imbalance (lack of estrogen). These same symptoms also can be caused by fluctuations in blood sugar. In numerous cases of what was first thought to be hormonal imbalance and estrogen deficiency, the solution was found not in taking hormones, but in stabilizing blood sugar levels.

Certainly hormonal imbalances can be caused by many things, including stress. But a big part of the problem has to do with something as seemingly innocuous as consuming a processed food snack, dessert or energy drink.

Eating too much white flour and sugar threatens our health.

When you eat a candy bar or drink a soda, blood sugar spikes. It doesn't take much; only a tablespoon or two of sugar is needed to do the trick. Too much sugar in the bloodstream is dangerous to the body. Over years of white flour and sugar consumption, the frequent high blood sugar surges can cause enormous free-radical damage, accelerating the aging process. In some people sugar can cause diabetes, resulting in heart disease, blindness, nerve damage, and brain cell death. The body knows this and acts to protect itself from high blood sugar by releasing the hormone insulin to store the excess sugar in the muscles, liver, and fat cells. That storage brings blood sugar down. When blood sugar then swings back downward, the body then steps in to release cortisol, the stress hormone, to keep blood sugar levels from getting too low. As we've already learned, excess production of cortisol ages the brain and puts stress on the adrenal gland, contributing to adrenal burnout. This so-called burnout makes it harder and harder for the gland to produce the stress-reducing hormones of testosterone (for men) and oxytocin (for women).

Excess blood sugar never used to be much of a dietary issue. When I was growing up, very few fast food restaurants or convenience stores existed. Today, though, the average person in America eats 100 times as much sugar as a person who lived a hundred years ago. Never before have so many empty calories, devoid of nutrition and packed with sugar, been available in people's diets. While this extra sugar gives us a boost of energy, it is also directly responsible for a host of problems, hormone deficiency being the most immediate.

Sugar in itself is not a bad food. It's an important fuel for the body and, in particular, the brain. Sugar only becomes a problem when we eat too much of it or if it's released too quickly into the bloodstream.

Let's use potatoes for an example. A baked potato converts immediately into sugar that floods into the bloodstream. Since this can easily be more sugar than the body needs, the excess sugar is stored as fat. This is why many weight-loss plans instruct dieters to avoid potatoes.

But we don't need to avoid potatoes. If you put a bit of butter or sour cream on your potato, the release of sugar into the bloodstream is slowed. Now there's no excess sugar to be stored as fat. As long as you aren't pre-diabetic, there are no negative effects to eating a potato combined with a bit of fat. Throughout history people have eaten buttered potatoes without becoming overweight.

I know it sounds complicated, but it's crucial to understand the basics of what happens when blood sugar levels fluctuate. Let's go through the steps once more:

1	You eat a couple of cookies made with white flour and corn syrup or sugar	Too much sugar is released into the bloodstream
2	Blood sugar rises	You feel a boost of energy
3	Insulin is released to store excess sugar	You get a little fatter
4	Blood sugar levels begin to drop	You want another cookie
5	Cortisol is released to stabilize blood sugar	Your adrenal gland becomes a little more exhausted and you feel miserable

Now it becomes clear why our hormone levels today are so low. Each time we eat a snack or meal made from processed foods, our body reacts with fluctuations in blood sugar which in turn raise cortisol levels. The effect is as if we're being chased by a bear all day long, every day. Our bodies are designed to handle stress very effectively, but not hour after hour, day after day. The adrenal gland becomes so busy producing cortisol that it can't keep up with the need for stress-busting hormones such as testosterone (for men) and oxytocin (for women.)

Let's look at how this plays out for a typical man and woman.

Woman: At the end of a stressful day, a woman who does recuperative things like talking about her feelings will make more serotonin to help her relax. If her blood sugar is low, however, she won't have the fuel for her brain to make serotonin and will begin to feel even more overwhelmed and stressed. She stops talking, but inside a monologue continues. She worries and over-thinks. With stable blood sugar, she would have the serotonin necessary to prevent this.

Man: To cope with stress, a man retreats to his cave. Resting helps him rebuild his testosterone levels, while a brain chemical called dopamine motivates him to come out of the cave. Dopamine is a brain hormone or neurotransmitter that increases feelings of pleasure, focus, and motivation. After a long day, a man runs out of dopamine and needs to find ways of making more. Reading the newspaper, solving a puzzle, meditating, and watching TV are common stimulators of dopamine. But if his blood sugar level is low, he can't make dopamine or testosterone. He goes into the cave and doesn't come out.

We see, once again, the difference in brain chemistry. Women tend to run out of serotonin while men tend to run out of dopamine. Serotonin allows her to relax and feel good while dopamine gives him the motivation to do things. Since women have a more active emotional center in the brain, they tend to run out of serotonin faster than do men. Men also have greater stores of serotonin because they make it 50 percent faster and store 50 percent more. But men don't have all the advantages: They tend to run out of dopamine faster than women. A man's greater muscle mass competes for the amino acids that make dopamine, so by the end of the day, a man has run out.

These brain-chemical differences can be the source of incompatibility and even conflict. At the end of a stressful day, a woman tends to have plenty of dopamine motivating her to get things done, but a shortage of serotonin. High dopamine tells her she has things to do and low serotonin tells her she has no time or support to get them done. She feels overwhelmed.

Meanwhile, a man comes home with low dopamine levels. He's not motivated to do anything, but he has plenty of feel-good serotonin allowing him to relax and rebuild his testosterone levels. He sees his stress melting away.

Mars and Venus are set up for collision. She's overwhelmed with too much to do and on fire because he's sitting on the couch, seemingly without a care in the world. He's on ice. As far as he is concerned, everything can be done tomorrow.

This imbalance of fire and ice would seem to be caused by a deficiency of feel-good brain chemicals. But there's a more basic cause: fluctuating blood sugar levels. If Mars and Venus can ensure themselves of a steady supply of blood sugar, women experience the immediate benefits of being able to talk about their day. And men, after some time in the cave, are ready to come out and join the living.

Blood Sugar on a Roller Coaster

We know that the main reason we have blood sugar problems is that we eat too many processed foods, along with foods and drinks that contain excessively high amounts of sugar. We must cut the sugar and eat more unprocessed foods if we want to enjoy stable blood sugar levels that allow our hormone factory, the adrenal gland, to produce feel-good hormones and reduce stress.

What's so good about unprocessed food? When foods aren't processed, the natural fiber in carbohydrates slows down the release of sugar into the bloodstream. Processed foods aren't good because sugar has been added and natural fiber has been removed. As a result, processed foods spike blood sugar. Almost everything in the center of the grocery store that is pre-packaged is a processed food deficient in natural fiber and containing added sugar. Almost everything at the perimeter of the store—produce, meat, fish, and some bread—is unprocessed and therefore healthier.

Bread and other baked goods are tricky. White bread or even whole wheat bread with "enriched wheat flour" is missing the whole grain that contains more fiber. The same is true of white rice. Fruit juices are less beneficial than it might seem, too, because they are devoid of the natural fiber of the whole fruit. In reality, fruit juice isn't much different than soda pop. Cookies, cakes, chips, pastries, doughnuts, pizza, and ice cream all lack the natural fiber that would normally slow down the release of sugar into the bloodstream. From the body's perspective, they offer only what we have far too much of: sugar.

Most people have little awareness of how much sugar is in the foods and drinks they consume. For example, a bottle of one of those vitamin-enriched water products sounds very healthy. Look at the label and it says 13 grams of sugar per serving. This doesn't sound too bad until you look above and discover that the bottle contains 2.5 servings. So, if you drink the whole bottle, you're getting 32.5 grams of sugar, or about eight teaspoons. Imagine putting eight teaspoons of sugar in your water and drinking it! If you did, you'd spike your blood sugar and later your adrenal gland would secrete cortisol, the stress hormone, to prevent your blood sugar from swinging back too low. In turn, you'd then have difficulty making the feel-good hormones and, as a result, mood swings are guaranteed.

You may wonder why people who have big swings in mood and energy don't necessarily show signs of low blood sugar when medically tested. There's a simple reason: Blood sugar tests may reveal diabetes (too much sugar) or chronic hypoglycemia (too little), but they don't reveal the fluctuations that affect most of us when we're not eating right. In reality, blood sugar doesn't have to be really low for you to feel hypoglycemic; it just has to be dropping rapidly from one moment to another. Just ask yourself: Do you have sugar or caffeine cravings? Do you experience low energy levels or mood swings one to three hours after a meal? If you answer "yes" to either question, you may be on the blood sugar roller coaster.

A personal observation: I used to experience intense anxiety before speaking to groups. But the anxiety went away when I stopped eating high amounts of sugar and completely avoided foods and drinks with sugar on the day of the event. For those who have a tendency toward anxiety, just reducing consumed sugar can help dramatically.

> Big mood swings can often be attributed to an overabundance of sugar and processed food in the diet.

Giving up sugar isn't easy. When we're under stress, sugar is wonderful fuel. Surely you've noticed that when you feel stressed, overwhelmed, bored or uncomfortable, you crave something sugary or something that turns immediately to sugar, like white rice, chips or bread. Once again, hormonal factors are at work. When both men and women aren't making enough anti-stress hormones, cortisol is released and the muscles stop burning fat for energy. Instead, they require sugar. When the muscles begin using up the sugar, there's not enough for the brain. That's why you're craving sugar.

But there's more. Remember that when cortisol levels spike, the body goes into emergency mode, as if being chased by a bear. Sugar provides quick energy like kindling wood. Fat provides long-lasting energy like a log. As long as we're eating too much sugar, our blood sugar fluctuates, raising cortisol levels, which causes us to crave ever more sugar. It's a vicious circle and we must intervene to stop it.

Addictions are difficult to overcome, but especially so when the addictive substance is something our bodies actually need. We don't need cigarettes or alcohol, but we do need sugar, in some form, every day.

Here's the cycle:
1. As stress levels go up, the body releases cortisol.
2. Elevated cortisol inhibits fat burning and stimulates sugar burning.
3. The muscles begin using up sugar.
4. Blood sugar levels begin to drop.
5. The brain orders you to eat more sugar.
6. More cortisol is released to stabilize fluctuating blood sugar levels.
7. The cycle begins again at step 2.

What's terribly unfair about this cycle is the recently discovered fact that just eating a candy bar with too much sugar can trigger the whole addictive cycle. That means that we don't need stress to stimulate the release of cortisol that then causes sugar cravings. Eating a candy bar can do the same. You could be completely stress-free when you decide to eat a candy bar with too much sugar, and your body will begin to react as if you're being chased by a bear. You feel good, but within a few hours your energy levels drop again.

So, how do we ensure that we get just the amount of sugar we need? By avoiding foods that are low in fiber and high in sugar. It sounds easier than it is. For example, white bread converts immediately into sugar. Taken without the fiber of a salad of raw vegetables, your blood sugar may fluctuate and you begin to crave more bread and thus overeat. By the end of the meal your blood sugar levels have dropped thanks to insulin stepping in to remove the excess sugar, so the dessert cart starts looking irresistible.

Stabilizing Blood Sugar Levels

Balancing blood sugar becomes easy if you're willing to follow an extremely healthy raw food diet free of all processed foods and sugars, but it's not an option for everyone. Fortunately there's an alternative, and it can be found in most health food stores.

Over the past 10 years, researchers at a variety of universities in Canada have developed and researched a new compound called PolyGlycopleX® (PGX®), a unique complex of water-soluble polysaccharides (plant fibers) that can help reduce blood sugar fluctuations. You simply take a few capsules or a small scoop of PGX® and a glass of water before meals and the results, supported by research, are amazing. I've never seen an all-natural product that can stabilize blood sugar as well as PGX®. There are lots of products available that can help, but this one is remarkable. I take it regularly and it has changed my life without requiring me to significantly change what I eat.

As I was getting into my 40s and 50s, I found myself getting sleepy after meals. I napped more, too. It was a gradual change and at first I thought little of it. But when I started taking PGX®, all that sluggishness stopped. I could eat pasta, bread, pizza, and desserts without those negative side effects. By using PGX® before meals and thus minimizing blood sugar fluctuations, I experienced sustained energy, much as I did as a younger man. Over the past two years, I have recommended PGX® to thousands of individuals and have received similar rave reviews.

Used before or with a meal, PGX® absorbs many times its weight in water within the digestive system. This action not only slows the absorption of carbohydrates (thereby slowing the release of sugar into the bloodstream), but allows you to reduce portion size while still feeling satisfied. Taking 2-5 grams of PGX® with meals helps prevent

PGX helps minimize fluctuations in blood sugar.

blood sugar from spiking after meals and helps get you off the blood sugar roller coaster once and for all. Not sure if you are riding the blood sugar roller coaster? See how many of these symptoms sound familiar:

- Waist is larger than hips
- Difficulty losing weight and keeping it off
- Craving sweets
- Feeling much better after you eat, only to feel awful a bit later
- Feeling irritable if you miss a meal
- Sometimes feeling a bit spacey, foggy or disconnected
- Elevated blood sugar or triglyceride levels
- Getting anxious for no apparent reason
- Waking up often during the night
- Feeling hungry all the time even when you know it's not time to eat
- Getting sleepy in the afternoon
- Craving caffeine or sugary drinks

In their book, *Hunger Free Forever,* Michael T. Murray, N.D., and Michael R. Lyon, M.D., describe how to use PGX® to stabilize blood sugar and tame your appetite for lifelong weight control. More energy, better sleep, improved memory and focus, increased motivation, stronger muscles, and automatic weight management are only a few of the immediate benefits of learning to balance your blood sugar.

By understanding how blood sugar fluctuations affect our cortisol levels, we can apply the information where it will do tremendous good: in the loving relationships of our lives. With a healthy body to support a healthy mind, we can then easily apply the Mars/Venus relationship insights to stimulate oxytocin and testosterone. In the next chapter we will explore new relationship skills for increasing romance. Women will find they get more of what they deserve from their men, and men will discover what they've been missing from their women!

CHAPTER 4

COOLING DOWN VENUS, HEATING UP MARS

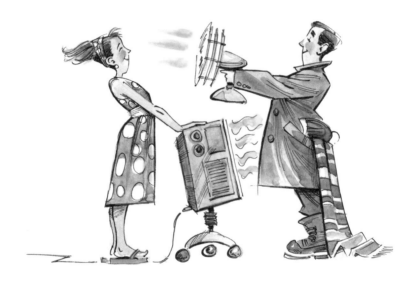

THE QUICKEST PATH TO THEIR HAPPINESS IS LOWERING THEIR STRESS LEVEL.

"Ladies first." It's true when opening a door, if you're a man with manners. It's also true when you're a hormone-savvy man seeking to improve his relationship with a woman.

Here's why: Couples tend to be only as happy as is the woman in the relationship. If she's under stress—and we've already shown that most women are more stressed-out than ever before—the quickest path to *his* happiness and *their* happiness is by lowering her stress level. In hormonal terms, it's like this: When a man finds ways of raising a woman's oxytocin level, thus lowering her stress level, it actually works to raise his testosterone level. And that increase in testosterone lowers his stress level, too.

In other words, everybody wins! The couple that seeks to restore the bliss of their courtship, or reach new heights in their domestic compatibility, must learn to think "woman first." It's her well-being that ensures the contentment of everyone around her.

Throughout this chapter I will frame much of my message for use by couples. But I invite you to look beyond my frame as you read. The insight you'll gain in this chapter is helpful even for those who think they're not in a relationship. The truth is that we are always in relationships with lots of people: parents, children, co-workers, friends, enemies, neighbors, past partners, and community members. Try some of my techniques in these other relationships and you may find that you don't have to be in love to make your interactions with others more loving.

Here's how we start: By understanding that virtually all the women we encounter are in hormonal deficit, whether they know it or not.

Let's look at this from a historical perspective. Before women began entering the workforce in large numbers, each female was surrounded by a community of other females, all of whom were engaged in the same sorts of nurturing activities. There were pluses and minuses to this type of lifestyle, but looking at it from a strictly hormonal perspective, it was advantageous to women. That's because their steady routine ensured that they always had enough oxytocin present in their systems to cope with stress.

But today, for all but the rare woman, oxytocin is in short supply. Modern women now shoulder far more testosterone-producing responsibilities than they used to. Instead of nurturing, they work at jobs that involve urgency or even emergency, along with problem solving and sacrifice. The extra testosterone generated by such jobs is a help when the job-holder is a man, because it reduces his stress level. But it doesn't help women. In fact, the surplus of testosterone and the relative deficiency of oxytocin leave many women frazzled and unhappy.

To effectively cope with stress, modern women need extra support. They need what I call *super-oxytocin producers*, present in their personal life to balance the many hours they spend making testosterone. Holding a job that stimulates testosterone production is fine—even great—as long as she can find enough opportunities to make oxytocin in her personal life. And men need to make it a priority to help her do that if they themselves are to be happy in their most important relationship.

Quality relationships and pleasurable activities are the make-or-break factors in the lives of today's women. To find balance and restore oxytocin levels, women must make time on a regular basis to do the things they enjoy, whether that's reading a good book, getting a manicure or a pedicure, taking the kids or grand-kids to the park, having lunch with a friend or getting away for a girls-only weekend. But scheduling fun can't become a new burden of responsibility or an act of desperation. Waiting until there's an urgent need, or getting goal-oriented about planning your super-oxytocin producers only gets you more testosterone! Think of your oxytocin stores as a bank account that benefits from regular deposits and regular withdrawals.

Women under stress tend to put their own needs at the end of their lengthy to-do list.

Of course this is easier said than done. Making time for themselves is not a priority for most women; in fact, women under stress, the ones who most need to avail themselves of super-oxytocin producers, are also the women who can't seem to fit their own needs onto their ever-lengthening list of things to do. They need help learning how to put themselves at the top of the list. This help can come from anyone, but a woman's ideal helper is the person closest to her, the man in her life.

Unfortunately, the average man has no idea how to help. That's not to say he's a fool. He knows, intuitively, that the most powerful super-oxytocin producer is romance. But that and a buck-and-a-half gets him bus fare—he really doesn't know what's romantic, and more importantly, he can't begin to guess what he can do that, *she will consider* romantic.

Before we get into the detail of that, I want to issue a bit of a caveat: The kind of romance most women think they're longing for tends to be impractical. In its most extreme form, a woman's unrealistic expectations can be described this way, "Romance is whenever he knows what I want even though I don't know what I need, but he supplies it without me having to ask." Whew. I'd rather go back to the couch and make some testosterone. Where's my remote?

This unrealistic romantic scenario, if played out, will certainly make a woman a lot of oxytocin, but it's rarely possible in real life. Maybe it happens in the movies, but not in any typical marriage.

Women don't always know what they want in romance, but they do know when they are not getting it.

How can he know what she wants, when quite often she herself doesn't even recognize it, much less express it? How many times does a man ask a woman where she wants to eat dinner and she says she has no idea... because she wants him to initiate and choose a romantic setting? He's lost. He doesn't know what to do. He just doesn't have the necessary information. And he resents being made to feel that he is to blame for her frustration.

A woman's need for romance is obvious to her, but how to go about getting it is not. It's nowhere near obvious to men how to provide it for her, either. Until the last several decades, it wasn't an issue men worried about. In my mother's generation and before, romance wasn't that important, at least not from a hormonal perspective. Back then a woman had her entire nurturing day to produce oxytocin, so she didn't need the super-oxytocin producers. Romantic gestures from a husband were definitely appreciated, but they weren't a necessity. A lack of romance certainly wasn't grounds for discontent.

Forty years ago or more, a woman had the time and the financial support to fill her day with an oxytocin-producing balance of nurturing and woman-to-woman support. Today's women enjoy the freedom of creating a career for themselves outside the home, but it has cost them the nurturing and support that rebuilds oxytocin and counteracts the testosterone they build up during a workday. It's ironic, but in a modern era in which women depend less on men—or not at all—they actually need men more than ever before. Women may not need men as providers and protectors as much as they once did, but if they want to maintain a healthy mind/body connection, they need a new kind of support from the opposite sex. Women need their men to help them stimulate super-oxytocin.

Creating a New Kind of Romance

Now let's look again at romance, this time from the perspective of getting women the oxytocin they need. On Venus, getting flowers stimulates oxytocin. A woman can buy them herself, and she should if she doesn't have someone to buy them for her! But, not surprisingly, getting flowers from a man is more fun for her. This is the difference between an oxytocin-producing activity and a super-oxytocin activity. It also defines for us that tricky word, romance: It's the little expressions of caring.

This could be news to the man in your life. When it comes to romance, men imagine something big and complicated. To them, romance is all the things they did in courtship to prove their love. And though there were little things on the list like flowers and chocolate, they probably focused more on the surprise birthday party, the tickets to a very special event, the carefully-planned marriage proposal. Women wonder, why did they stop doing these things? Well, in the minds of men, they haven't stopped! A man concludes, "Now that I'm doing the big things like working to provide for her, I don't need to do all that other stuff. Besides, she does most of the shopping, so if she wants flowers, why can't she pick them up while she's at the grocery store?"

This is completely logical and utterly wrong. Many men just don't understand that little things that say, "I care" matter deeply to women. That's because they can't relate. While small gestures stimulate oxytocin and reduce stress in women, they aren't the sorts of things that would make any sort of dent in a man's stress.

Men who want to stimulate super-oxytocin in their women must get past the idea that bigger is better. This is counterintuitive to many of them. They think, "If I do something big, it'll pay off big." So, gentlemen, remember that when it comes to super-oxytocin, it's not how big but how many. If you bring her three dozen roses, you might think you'll make 36 points with her. But on Venus the scoring system is different. You get one point for every act of love, no matter how big or small. Remember that: One point per act of love. Bigger is not better, but more is. If you want to score 36 points, you need to bring *one* rose... *36 times.*

> Numerous small gestures of love count for more on Venus than one big event.

Of course, this isn't a man-only task, this romance business. Women can be just as clueless as men in this area. For example, a man could take his wife out to dinner, only to hear her spend half the evening talking about how various dishes could be improved. To her it's just conversation, and if she were sitting there with a woman, it would be exactly that, and it would produce oxytocin for both of them! But to a man, such topics sound like complaining. You see, on a romantic date, a man needs to hear messages of success, because feeling successful stimulates his stress-reducing production of testosterone. This is just as important to him as feeling cared for is to her. He needs to hear that his woman is enjoying the experience, because he can then feel proud and happy that he provided her a wonderful evening out.

Here's another way in which women don't make it easy for their men: Too many women expect their men to do it all, romantically speaking, and when the men try but fall short, the women are disappointed—and show it. Women need to take their share of responsibility. Instead of making him play a guessing game, a woman needs to let her man know what she would like and, *ask him to provide it.* That's right; to ensure that she gets the super-oxytocin she needs, her job is to know what she wants and make the request. His job is to say yes and deliver.

This scenario packs a double benefit. Asking for what she wants and being assured of getting it gives a woman an oxytocin boost for however many days she anticipates the delivery of the romantic gesture she requested. That boost offsets the testosterone she makes on the job and leaves her happier and less stressed. And, when the magic day arrives, it's a super-oxytocin producer for her, because her small dream has come true at the hands of the man she loves. And as we know, when a woman is happy, so is her man.

Men need motivation in romance, just as in other things they do. To keep a man motivated to provide super-oxytocin producers, a woman doesn't have to offer a standing ovation. She must simply appreciate the things he does. In essence, romance is created when he repeats the little things he did in the beginning of their relationship, and she, in turn, re-creates the delight and appreciation she felt back then.

Let's take a few moments to think about how things worked when love was new, so we can understand what we need to do to rekindle some of that passion.

Stimulating the Hormones of Love and Desire

In the beginning of a relationship there isn't much we have to do to stimulate the hormones of love and desire. Just the newness of having a relationship stimulates these heavenly hormones and motivates us to act and respond in romantic ways. Hormonally speaking, boy meets girl and dopamine levels in the brain rise, helping to increase the male testosterone levels that lead to sexual attraction. Women respond with higher levels of serotonin, motivating them to give freely—which, in turn, stimulates the release of super-oxytocin. Ah, bliss.

But newness wears off. After the rosy glow of courtship has faded we must depend on mutual understanding and good relationship skills to sustain the romantic feelings. This is often difficult for couples, because they remember that romance was once automatic, and so they expect it to always be that way. It can't be. There's no newness to stimulate the dopamine production anymore. We must find new ways of getting our feel-good hormones made. We need to work purposefully to make it happen.

Here's the key knowledge we need, in an easy-to-recall phrase: *Just as hormones stimulate actions and attitudes... actions and attitudes stimulate hormones.* By simply repeating the romantic actions and responses we experienced in the beginning of a relationship we can bring back the romantic feelings. This important strategy works for men and women in different ways.

Even if he's not in a romantic mood, if a man makes the effort to take action—a kiss, a squeeze—these small moves will raise his testosterone levels, and he'll feel great. When a woman makes moves to be romantic, it will also increase her testosterone level. But this does little for her oxytocin levels. Indeed, when women persist in trying to do more for their partners, they often end up feeling used and resentful.

So, a woman must go at it from a different direction. A woman can best increase her romantic feelings by focusing on her attitude and not her actions. By trying to be more loving in her responses to her partner, she will increase her oxytocin production and lower her stress levels. Taking time to reflect on and appreciate all that her partner provides for her will not only lower her stress levels but also empower him to do more for her.

This concept of creating the hormones of romance by acting and responding in a romantic manner seems awkward to some people. They presume that romance should be spontaneous, not planned. That's because romance was spontaneous in the beginning. But once spontaneity is gone it doesn't come back unless we do something to bring it back. Fortunately, there's a lot we can do, but it takes deliberate intention. Let's explore an example of this:

In the beginning of a relationship, because the hormone releases are automatic, a man will spontaneously create a plan to please his partner. But when the hormones are no longer automatic, this same man just doesn't feel like planning a date. It's much easier to wait until the weekend and ask his partner what she'd like to do. This may seem loving, at least to him, but it's actually very passive and will eventually kill the passion in a relationship. Planning special times together is an important ingredient of romance. Our aim is... a man with a plan, and a woman with a smile.

It takes plenty of testosterone to make a husband into a man with a plan. It takes plenty of oxytocin to keep a smile on a woman's face. But, as we pointed out in the beginning of this chapter, it's "ladies first"; her feelings matter most when the goal is the return of romance. If a man can get past everything that stops him from making a plan—fatigue, inertia, past disappointments—and just goes ahead and does it, he'll see his woman smile. He will also see his stress evaporate. Yes, planning dates actually produces testosterone and reduces stress!

Women love a man with a plan just as men love a woman with a smile!

A man should think of this as a requirement of his husbandly job. Think of this: At work a man doesn't think twice about doing things he doesn't "feel" like doing. He does them because it's necessary to get the job done. His reasoning goes, "I don't want to do it, but if it's necessary, I'm happy to do it." This is the same thinking he ought to apply to his relationship. If he wants to keep the passion and attraction alive, he must do certain things that have been proven to work, even if at first he doesn't feel like it.

Women, too, have an inertia barrier to overcome. Under stress and lacking sufficient oxytocin, a woman may think she's too overwhelmed to go out on a date. But if she allows a man to plan it for her, she'll find that she begins to relax and feel happy. By allowing him to take care of her, instead of her taking care of him, her oxytocin levels gradually go up and she begins to smile again. She may not love the movie or restaurant he chose, but she *will* love that he took the initiative to make the date and try to meet her needs.

The thing to keep in mind, for both men and women, is that what we once did automatically to create romance is now, too often, something we unconsciously resist.

1. Our resistance to sharing

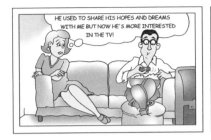 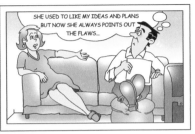

2. Our resistance to romance

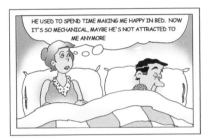 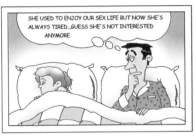

3. Our resistance to needing each other

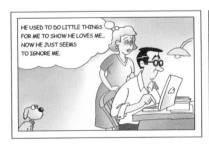 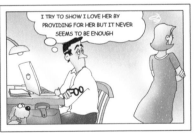

4. Our resistance to talking

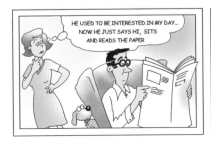 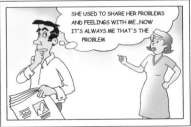

5. Our resistance to opening up

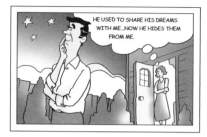 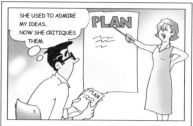

6. Our resistance receiving help

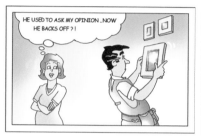 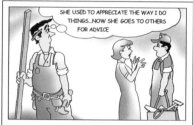

7. Our resistance to caring

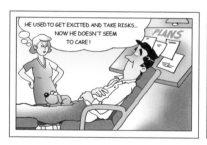 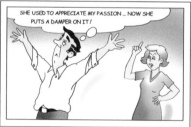

8. Our resistance to passion

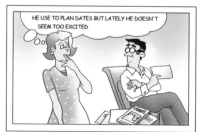 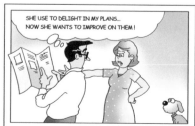

What we see in the previous boxes is the effect of increasing stress and a failure of the mind/body connection. As time goes on and relationships mature, both men and women who aren't getting their stress levels reduced by sufficient production of stress-busting hormones start acting in ways that only make things worse. Men become more passive. Women become more demanding. Mars and Venus drift ever further apart.

What can we do to bring back the good feelings that came so automatically when romance was new? We can teach ourselves how to get what we need.

Achieving Lasting Romance and Passion

It might seem that the simplest solution for stressed-out couples would be to remember what worked in the beginning and just start doing it again. If it made you happy in the past, it will make you happy in the future.

Unfortunately, no. Creating romance is like climbing into a bath. If the water's warm, you can turn on the jets and enjoy the warmth. But if the water is cold to begin with, turning on the jets isn't going to improve your comfort. A new relationship is like a warm bath in the beginning that cools over time. Once the newness is gone, we have to find a way to warm the water again. It takes subtle shifts in thinking, simple changes in how we relate to one another.

> Once the newness is gone, we need to find new ways to warm the heart and restore the magic of romance.

Years ago, before we had the scientific understanding of hormones and how they differ in men and women and how we relate to one another, I could only tell people what to say and do to improve their relationship with the opposite sex. I based it on my own experiences and discoveries, and it worked for thousands of personal clients and the readers of my books. But what a difference it makes for us to have this hormonal understanding backing us up all the way! Many things that didn't make sense before begin to make sense now. The differences in our hormonal needs give rise to a multitude of insights to help explain the many mysteries of the opposite sex. It may take a lifetime for men to fully understand women and vice-versa, but with our new knowledge, we stand to become much closer much faster. If we're patient, we can gradually come to understand the biochemically-based reasons our partners act and react the way they do.

With understanding comes new perspective. What used to be annoying in your partner can become lovably humorous. Things that used to bruise egos and hurt feelings can be seen as simply words or gestures taken the wrong way. Instead of feeling frustration or helplessness in our attempts to communicate our love as well as our needs, we see the hope of achieving greater clarity and openness in the years ahead.

Before we go deeper into the ways we can use our newfound grasp of the mind/body connection to improve our relationship, let me share a small example of how my hormone-based understanding of Mars and Venus helps me relate better to Bonnie, my wife:

Recently Bonnie casually mentioned she was getting her hair cut and colored the next day. If I didn't understand women and their hormonally-based needs, I would have wondered why she told me. From a purely Martian perspective, it's, "Who cares if she's getting her hair cut?"

Now I know why she told me and why I should care. She told me she was getting her hair cut so that I would notice it on my own and comment, which I did a day later. This didn't come naturally; it was something I had to learn. Men rarely care if their Martian friends notice their haircut and they certainly don't ask anybody if they noticed! Believe me, the words, "Did you notice my haircut?" and, "What do you think of the new color?" have rarely been spoken on Mars. On Venus it's a different story; haircuts, hair color, makeup, outfit, sales, shoes, and accessories are all big topics of discussion.

Now, because I understand Venus a little better, I recognize that women give men hints all the time to help us be successful in providing what they need. Changing things like outfits and hair color are subtle hints saying, "Notice me." If a woman has to ask, "How do I look?" it's definitely not oxytocin-producing. No matter what his response, it wouldn't create the warm feelings that occur when a man, on his own, notices a change and compliments her. So, don't make her have to ask! Watch and listen for the clues.

Remember, "Ladies first." A man's mission is to make himself happier by making his woman happier. The warmth she feels when her man notices and appreciates her is an indicator to both partners that she's producing oxytocin and relieving her stress. Because little compliments have nowhere near the same effect on men, men underestimate their value. To understand the magnitude of such a small act, men ought to imagine how they would feel when complimented... and multiply it 10 times! The same goes for being ignored: However bad it feels to him, he should multiply it 10 times for her.

But, as always, women have a role to play in this duet. Because testosterone doesn't lower stress in a woman's body she doesn't instinctively understand what a big difference it makes to him when she appreciates what he does—or when she doesn't focus on what he didn't do! When a woman overlooks a man's mistake, he may not say anything, but he definitely notices. The rule of 10x applies again: His pleasure is at least 10 times greater than hers because he needs testosterone so much more. His pain is also 10 times greater when she gives him messages that are critical. This ought to explain why men are somewhat resistant to a woman's suggestions of how to do something. Her attempt to change or improve him can easily sound like lack of trust or appreciation.

Women need to realize that if a man doesn't notice her new haircut, either he doesn't understand the importance of oxytocin-producing events or he's under stress and has completely forgotten. In both cases he's clueless, and for her to resent him for it is just a waste of energy. You can't make a man be more like a woman.

> Women enjoy getting compliments. Men enjoy being appreciated for what they do.

He and she are biochemically different. And knowing this makes it easier for her not to take things so personally.

Still, this doesn't mean that a woman must give up her needs. A woman should have girlfriends to do the noticing and commenting. She should also ensure that she's giving herself enough super-oxytocin producers to keep her supply of feel-good hormones filled to the brim. Women who find ways of ensuring that other areas of their lives fill them to 90 percent—leaving just 10 percent for their men to fill—find that they're happy. And they're often amazed at how their happiness can transform their men into much more attentive and supportive partners. It's not magic; it's our heavenly hormones at work, acting and interacting on our mind/body connection.

Happiness is a two-way street. When I feel good, my wife seems to blossom before my eyes. And when she feels good, it becomes so easy for me to give her the attention and support she so much appreciates from me. The better we both feel, the better is our relationship. Falling in love years ago was wonderful, but it only gave us a glimpse of what was possible in the relationship. It takes a lifetime to fully manifest the vision.

Hormones Make All the Difference

I hope it's now clear that giving our partners what we ourselves might want is often the opposite of what will work. Certainly on many levels men and women are just the same—we all want to be safe, happy, successful and loved. But what we need to feel this way can be very different, thanks to our hormonal differences.

Let's zero in on a couple of examples:

Achievement: Whatever makes a man feel successful and thus raises his testosterone levels will capture his attention and give him energy. Women certainly want respect for their actions and achievements, but the acknowledgement itself is not a big stress reducer. Women often wonder why men make such a big deal out of taking credit for things. This is simply because taking credit stimulates testosterone. Women don't readily relate to the importance of receiving credit because testosterone doesn't lower a woman's stress levels. But when a man makes it easy for a woman to get the support she needs to achieve, especially without being asked, her oxytocin levels go up, and she responds lovingly and appreciatively.

Assistance: Men don't like being offered help unless they ask for it. To offer help to a guy with a problem may imply that you think he can't solve it himself. A man's sense of self-esteem is centered around what he can do. This is because it's the success of his actions and the wisdom of his decisions that increases his testosterone levels. Getting help stimulates oxytocin, which does nothing to lower his stress levels. A woman, though, is much more open to asking for this kind of support, and the oxytocin created reduces her stress. When someone offers to help her, it can put a big smile on her face. On Venus it's the quality of relationships that counts much more than how successful any one Venusian

> Giving our partners what we might want is often the opposite of what they need.

may be. In hormonal terms, the oxytocin produced from doing things with others is much more important to a woman than the testosterone produced by doing things on her own.

You know the old saw about men never asking for directions? Or the true fact that men tend to put off going to a doctor? Hormonal differences explain these things beautifully.

When I ask men in my seminars if they stop and get directions, most of them will say they do. Their women laugh in disbelief. The truth is that men do ask for directions—they just do it when their partners aren't around! When in the car, she senses that he needs help long before he does. This only adds extra motivation for him to prove to her that he's not lost.

Something similar happens with help-seeking. A man will ask for medical and other sorts of assistance, but only after he feels he's done everything he can on his own. Then, asking for help can be testosterone-producing because it becomes the way he's solving the problem. His timing is just different from a woman's.

Bringing Back the Romance

With these comparisons and contrasts as background, I want to return once more to the ways we can use our hormonal knowledge and improved relationship skills to bring romance back into our lives post-courtship. This also takes us back to "Ladies first."

By choosing to take romantic action even when he's not feeling automatically motivated, a man gets the right hormones flowing so he can feel the romance again. By choosing to respond in ways that she did in the beginning of the relationship, a woman's romantic feelings are rekindled. It's the old saying, "Fake it until you make it." But we're not really faking it. We're simply taking action or expressing our feelings to more fully experience the love that we know is in our hearts.

The important point here is that a man must first take action before a woman can choose to respond in a positive and appreciative manner. If he's not taking action—or if she's the only one who has read this book—she'll need to ask for what she wants. When he responds, she too can respond.

If asking feels difficult, a woman can start the process by writing in her journal every day for a week about what her partner provides that she appreciates. If she can't easily reflect on 10 or 20 things, she should first write out all the things she doesn't like about her life. After about 10 minutes of that, she'll become more aware of what she does like. Asking for more of it shouldn't be difficult.

> Men need to hear clear, friendly and direct requests instead of complaints.

One of the biggest obstacles to lasting romance is that women feel a variety of wants, wishes and needs, but they don't share them with their partners. This is a dangerous disconnection in a relationship. If a woman isn't asking for what she wants, a man will assume she must be getting what she wants already.

To avoid such misunderstandings, men need to hear clear, friendly and short requests. Then, when he responds to her requests, she can practice giving him the kind of support she gave in the beginning of the relationship. By doing this, she'll be helping him feel romantic and more connected to her, and she'll be getting the kind of attention she finds so hard to ask for. If he shows no interest in responding to her request, she should simply wait and try again in a few days as if she's asking for the first time. This helps a woman not feel like she is nagging, and it has the same effect on the man.

If a woman complains about what she's not getting instead of asking for what she wants, the man won't feel like being romantic. On Mars, it's almost impossible to feel romantic when someone is complaining that you're not doing enough. Remember, it is success—not failure—that stimulates testosterone levels. Instead of pointing out his mistakes or correcting him, she can focus on appreciating even the littlest thing he does for her, just as she did in the past. Believe me, it will pay dividends.

Here are some examples of ways that women can ask for romance. Try these, but always remember that you must practice showing appreciation for what you get from your man, instead of focusing on what you're not getting:

- "This is going to be a great concert. Would you get tickets and plan a date for us?"

- "We've been invited to a party. I know you don't like parties much, but would you come as my fabulous date?"

- "I had such a long day. Would you make reservations and take me out to dinner?"

- "I got my hair colored today. Did you notice? I like it a lot. You, too?"

- "There's a great play coming and I got tickets. Would you put it on your calendar and take me?"

- "Well, how do I look? I know you always think I look pretty good, but it feels good to hear it."

- "The weather is supposed to be great this weekend. Let's hang out at the shore on Saturday, shall we? I'll make a picnic and you can drive."

- "I'm worn out. Would you take care of the dishes tonight?"

- "I finally have some time to focus on cleaning the garage. Would you help me with it this weekend?"

- "Sometimes I miss hearing you say you love me. I know you do, but it's nice to hear you say it. Would you surprise me with it now and then?

As you can see, each of these requests is direct, brief and positive. She doesn't complain or dredge up old issues to justify asking for his support. By using just a few words, she makes it easier for him to take action and give her the answer she is hoping for.

By taking the "Ladies first" road to mutual happiness, and then working together to deliberately do some of the romantic things you used to do, Venus and Mars can discover that they have the power to endlessly renew their own good feelings and retain the spark that brought them together. Our growing understanding of the simple changes and subtle shifts it takes to stimulate the stress-reducing, feel-good hormones is what makes it all possible.

In the next chapter we will discuss how—yikes!—Mars and Venus can actually find themselves reversing roles. We'll talk about how partners can lovingly relate when men and women find themselves having switched places.

CHAPTER 5

VENUS AND MARS, CHANGING PLACES?!?

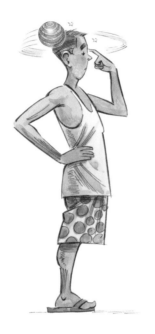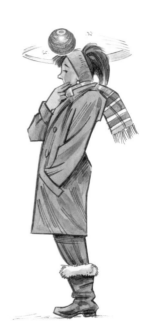

ROLE REVERSAL—THE RESULT OF
A RELATIONSHIP THAT HAS GOTTEN
OUT OF BALANCE.

While most men and women can relate to the characterizations of Mars on Ice and Venus on Fire, there are some for whom the labels don't fit. With more women in the workplace being rewarded for their ability to think and behave like men, it's becoming increasingly common for some women to wonder which planet they're really from. They begin to wonder about their husbands, too!

With elevated levels of testosterone and not enough oxytocin, a woman will sometimes begin to feel that *she* is the one from Mars, and that her man surely must have a Venusian birth certificate. In my experience, a deeper look will always reveal the truth—that she really is from Venus and he really is from Mars, and their place-switching is just an indication of a relationship gone out of balance. But on the surface, it can certainly seem like the role reversal is for real. And that's what makes it worth talking about in this chapter.

As women shoulder more responsibilities that traditionally belonged to men, men will automatically move more to their Venusian side, with undesirable results. Just as women who move too much to their masculine side become overwhelmed with too many testosterone-producing duties and not enough nurture-derived oxytocin to reduce stress, men moving too much to their female side will become more passive, needy, and testosterone-poor. Too often, communication between the two breaks down and romance dies.

Does role reversal mean that the Mars-woman quits shopping or wanting to talk? Actually, no. As I've said, deep down, she's still from Venus. These Mars-women still act like Venusians when they're on their own time in a non-work world. But at home she's made herself a cave, she's retreating to it nightly, and suddenly her desire to talk is far exceeded by her partner's!

What Causes Role Reversal?

In some cases, role reversal is a learned behavior from childhood. If a girl grows up in a family where feelings are ridiculed or pushed aside, she'll learn to suppress this feminine part of her. Similarly, if a boy grows up in a family where masculinity is destructive, then, without a positive role model he will either bond more with his mother and become less masculine, or go the other way and become more macho. I call that the dark side of Mars.

But, often, role reversal is simply the result of a relationship that has gotten out of balance. As always, hormones play a role. When Venus becomes Mars and vice-versa, it's because neither party in the relationship is doing the things needed to release and restore the biochemical substances that assure the health of their mind/body connection.

Let's zero in on what the woman does in role reversal, because as we've seen, her happiness or unhappiness has far more impact on her love relationship than his will ever have.

When Women Become Cave Dwellers

Going to her cave is one of the most common and telltale signs of a woman who mistakenly thinks she's from Mars. Returning home from work, she withdraws—and *he's* the one who stands at the cave door trying to draw her out, because—get this—he wants to talk! You'd think that would be a welcome change to his wife, but it definitely is not. She doesn't want to talk and she doesn't want to listen. She wants to be alone.

Why doesn't she want to share with her partner? Because when she talks, she finds that he doesn't listen to her. With no way to share feelings and be heard, she copes with her frustration by shutting down communication. In effect, she has disconnected herself from her natural need for oxytocin. She's gone Martian. And, her man responds by taking on a more Venusian role.

Women stop talking when they don't trust they will be fully heard.

Remember, it's feeling heard that releases oxytocin and lowers stress for women. When she's out of balance and acting Martian, she's convinced that she won't be heard, so why should she bother sharing her feelings? She may even believe that sharing her feelings is a waste of her time. This isn't because she truly is from Mars, but because she is a Venusian who has gotten herself stuck. She doesn't even understand that her true need is to be heard, so she doesn't seek out ways to be heard. Instead, she isolates herself and feels increasingly overwhelmed by her work and her unrelieved stress.

Has she fallen out of love? No. But she's not getting what she wants and needs, and she loathes the way her man is responding to her. He seems to have forgotten how to stimulate testosterone for himself in a healthy way, because he doesn't go to his cave anymore. All he seems to do is boast to her about his accomplishments or complain about his rotten day. None of this relieves her stress and, oh, does she have stress.

When Mars is on fire and Venus is on ice in this way, things are bad in the relationship and, many times, trying to make things better seems only to make things worse. But there's good news! There are ways to, well, reverse the role reversal and bring the relationship back into balance. In this chapter we'll take a look at the power of re-establishing the proper sorts of **talking, giving, and pleasing** for each gender. By subtly redirecting interactions in these areas, we find that both parties return to making their feel-good hormones. They also return to having reasonable expectations of one another and their relationship together. The woman returns to Venus, and the man goes back to Mars.

But before we get into solutions, let's spend a little time looking at things from the man's point of view.

When Men Talk Too Much

What's the story on the men? Why aren't they taking cave time for themselves? More importantly, why are their women in the cave instead?

In my experience, these men are needy, and it's their neediness that pushes their partners away. These are men who tend to do a lot around the house because their wives are busy, but the men aren't happy about it. They've grown picky and demanding and so insecure that they act self-impressed. When such a man talks he's not just sharing feelings, he's either trying to pump himself up by bragging or gain pity by whining. But he doesn't understand that his approach is a turn-off to his partner.

Let me stop here to dispel a common misconception. Being from Mars doesn't mean you don't talk. In the work world, men quite often talk much more than women! That's because men display dominance and authority by being talkative. When a man comes home and talks more than the woman does, it's not about sharing. It's usually so he can prove himself right about something. To cope with stress, he'd be better off taking cave time and learning to at least temporarily forget his problems instead of complaining about them. But instead he talks.

> Men talk to brag, self-justify, or misguidedly, to cope.

Show me a man who likes to talk a lot and I'll show you a man paired with a woman who doesn't talk. Whenever this role reversal takes place, it's bound to be a coping mechanism for both parties. Somewhere along the way he felt encouraged to talk about his problems, and she was discouraged from talking about hers. He feels her pulling away when he talks, so he talks more to try to re-engage her. She becomes even more annoyed, and pulls further away.

Ultimately, to find balance, a Venusian man needs to examine himself and take cave time to cope effectively with his stress. If he needs to talk more, he should do that—with his friends. With his partner, he should present himself as a listener.

There are reasons why his woman shouldn't be his sounding board. At the end of the day, she has little to give him. He needs to cope with his stress on his own and then offer his support to his woman in ways that will really make a hormonal difference. A good rule for men to remember in personal relationships is, *never talk more than the woman does.* Instead, a man seeking to prevent or correct role reversal should spend his time doing a variety of things designed to stimulate her oxytocin production. As we've seen in previous chapters, that won't only help her. It will make him feel good as well. And feeling good is the first step toward getting both partners back into their appropriate roles.

> A good rule for a man to remember is to make sure he never talks more than his woman.

Having worked with thousands of couples, I find that Mars-Venus role reversal is much more common in couples that have long-standing difficulties, and its prevalence increases the longer these men and women stay together. Still, it doesn't take years of therapy or relationship counseling to correct this situation; the parties involved just need to learn better ways of relating. At the same time they must come to really understand why a different set of interactions will improve the biochemical basis of their relationship. Then it's practice, practice, practice. At first some of the corrections will feel unnatural and maybe even forced. But with time and repetition, it all becomes second nature. That's because these techniques are harmoniously balanced with the differing effects of their male and female hormones.

Talking, Giving, and Pleasing

Now let's set the stage for understanding the three categories of improved interaction—talking, giving, and pleasing. Each of these is a key factor in a healthy relationship, and each is also an area prone to problems that lead to and perpetuate role reversal.

We need to ensure that both men and women are playing their gender-specific parts in these interactions, especially when the planets have switched orbits.

Before we go any further, please know that I'm not trying to undo decades of social progress here. Respecting gender tendencies doesn't imply that a woman can't be a Ms. Fix-It around the house, or that men can't be cooks or stay-at-home parents. It only means that in order to cope with the stresses of daily life they must take steps to stimulate their own gender-specific stress-reducing hormones.

A quick refresher before we go on: The more women take on male roles in the workplace, the less oxytocin they make. Likewise, the more men take on female roles, the less testosterone they make. This, by now, should be basic to you. You also know that women restore their oxytocin by nurturing and/or receiving support for their nurturing. Men restore their testosterone by taking up residence—daily but temporarily, we hope—in the cave. And all of this can work just fine even when partners are functioning in nontraditional roles.

Consider David and Beth. David, a stay-at-home parent, cares for the children while his wife, a professional chiropractor, is the major breadwinner. Variations of this pattern exist across the nation today. David's job as home parent would be totally exhausting if he failed to take time for himself away from the family by exercising in the gym, riding his bike or playing sports. For him, working out is a way he can express his masculinity and rebuild his testosterone levels.

> Respecting gender tendencies doesn't imply that women shouldn't use a wrench and men shouldn't be cooks.

David's wife, Beth, encourages him to go off and do what he needs to do because she knows he needs to balance all the nurturing he does with plenty of testosterone-releasing and -replacing activities. If she finds that David, who spends his days on his female side, wants to talk when she gets home, Beth wisely discourages him. She tells him something that may sound odd, but is on the mark for respecting gender differences in the household: She tells him to talk with his friends, and when he feels better, he should then come home and listen to her talk!

Beth, too, looks to her personal friendships to get a lot of the female support she needs for creating oxytocin. With David, she schedules time for romance, and also time for her feelings to be heard by him. It may sound selfish of Beth to do things this way, but she's a smart woman. She knows that this approach satisfies her need for oxytocin and David's need for testosterone.

Remember, when things go haywire, it's because the woman is too testosterone-laden from her work to recognize that she's not feeling heard. Often, she's paired with a man who doesn't know how to listen. Whether it's because he likes to hear himself talk or he can't stop himself from offering solutions, the result is the same: Women shut down. It's Venus on ice, exactly the opposite of the fiery place she should be. She finds herself doing the things people do on the red planet, like hanging out in the cave.

But a woman's Venus cave is not a man cave. A man cave is for coping with the outside world. A Venus cave is for isolating a woman from just one person—her partner. Why does she need to exclude him? Because, to her, he's just one more person who has nothing to give and plenty to take. She's been giving all day. She has nothing left.

For her, there's no point in talking or sharing feelings. Having lacked experience in sharing words and emotions to lower stress, she feels an even greater compulsion to stay stuck on her male side, the one that wants to solve problems. Having too much to do, she views talking as a complete waste of time. That's because she's never tasted the fulfillment of being fully heard as a way of coping with stress.

So, I hope you're seeing two things: First, that David and Beth, with their nontraditional yet very gender-oriented ways of doing things, have managed to avoid all the conflict I've just described. Second, please notice that unrelieved stress is at the heart of most role reversal.

When there is tension between men and women, he will become Mars on Fire and she will become Venus on Ice. This role reversal occurs generally because he hasn't learned how to manage his frustrations by temporarily forgetting them. That's how men are designed to cope with stress. If he doesn't know how to put his troubles out of mind, he will feel a compulsion to talk about them, thus pulling him out of his Martian role. It may feel good to him to talk, but it does little to help him effectively cope with stress.

On the other hand, she hasn't learned how to fully feel and express what's inside of her. She buries her feelings and feels compelled to always do more. Unable to most effectively cope with stress, she's more overwhelmed and has no time or is too exhausted for talking about feelings. Gradually these women become ever more like men and ever more disconnected from their softer, feminine side. The change in the mind makes a change in the body: These Mars-women often begin experiencing physical manifestations of hormone deficiency, led by an increasing inability to sleep at night and symptoms of premenstrual syndrome (PMS).

Interestingly enough, the solution for a couple experiencing role reversal is exactly the same as when things are where they belong and Venus is on Fire and Mars is on Ice. She needs to learn how to share her feelings so he'll listen, and he needs to learn how to stop interrupting and do some active listening as she expresses her feelings. Returning from role reversal is like walking a tightrope: Balance is imperative. If you start to wobble to the left or right, you work to find the balance point. When men are listening and seeking to understand—and women are sharing and feeling more understood—the balance point is found and restored.

Getting Men and Women What They Need

In my experience everyone thinks they know what they need. But if they're not getting their needs fulfilled, it's generally because they're looking in the wrong direction. If they really knew what they needed, wouldn't it be easy to get it?

When couples come to me for counseling they're almost always looking at solutions that won't work. Women often want men to talk, when their real need is to be heard. Men want to correct how women feel, when their real need is to change their approach so they can feel successful in supporting them. Women want men to change when really they need to find a way to change how they respond to situations. Men want women to be more responsive sexually when really they need to be more responsive to their women's romantic needs. Women often want men to open up and share their feelings when what they really need is for themselves to open up and share more of their feelings. In this case the man does not need to share more but to learn how to become a better listener so that he can make it safer for her to open up.

For the remainder of the chapter I'll attempt to cut through the misconceptions and offer a bit of a tutorial for couples seeking to achieve or restore balance.

One of the most powerful ways to restore hormonal balance in a relationship is, of course, romance. But at a certain point in an unbalanced relationship, efforts to create romance just bring more of the stress the couple is unable to relieve. This is especially true if the couple is under the mistaken impression that what worked at the beginning of the relationship can still work. As we saw in the last chapter, that's a fallacy. Once the newness is gone, romance is no longer automatic and must be stimulated by the good feelings of relieving each other's stress. You simply can't feel loving if you're not feeling good.

Do you remember that in the last chapter I encouraged marital partners to get 90 percent of what they need from the world and just 10 percent from the man or woman they love? Now I'm going to say more about why: Think of one of those fund-raising events where they put up a thermometer to indicate progress toward a goal. As more and more people donate, the red line on the thermometer moves up the scale from 10 percent to 20 percent and so on,

Romance corrects role reversal, but only if you're feeling good.

until the goal is reached at 100 percent. In your relationship, once the newness is gone, your romantic relationship can only move the thermometer of fulfillment 10 percent—from the 90 percent mark to 100 percent. Your own efforts and choices, independent of your romantic partner, are what raise the first 90 percent. After that, it's your partner's romantic donations that can, and do top the chart.

So that's key. Mars and Venus resume their own orbits when a series of changes occur, starting with *feeling good*.

To raise your thermometer of fulfillment and ensure balance in your relationship, you must cultivate areas of support in your life that don't involve your partner. You must find newness, hope, challenge and optimism in other areas of your life. That's how you get to 90 percent. At that point it's easy for your romantic relationship to take you and your partner from the 90 percent level of feeling good to the 100 percent level of feeling great! It is then, and only then, that you can make the changes that will restore Mars and Venus to their proper orbits.

Correcting Course

When an airplane takes off and flies on automatic pilot, it will almost certainly arrive at its destination. The course it takes may seem perfect, but it's not. At some point on its route, due to changing wind speeds and other factors, it's actually off course. But it's generally moving in the right direction. What it takes to keep it on course is nothing more than a series of small adjustments.

Course correction is how we keep relationships in balance, too. Ideally, we adjust for one another's gender-based differences with a clear-eyed acceptance of the fact that what works for him is not likely to work for her, and vice-versa. Without an understanding of each other's different needs, men and women are constantly adjusting and correcting their actions and reactions to no avail. Without an understanding of our differences, we may tend to follow our instincts. And our instincts, unfortunately, too often drive us further off course.

Indeed, our time-honored practice of following our instincts is dangerous, especially in the areas of *talking* to one another, *giving* to one another and *pleasing* one another. In each case, we *think* we know each other's modus operandi, but we probably don't. Let's consider them in reverse order and see if we can gain some mutual understanding.

Pleasing One Another

The perfect partner for a man is a woman he can please. In his ideal world, when he returns home each day he feels confident that he's meeting her expectations and fulfilling her desires.

A man's desire to make a woman happy is often underappreciated by women. She doesn't understand, because women have such different motivations. Certainly both are motivated to be happy together, but a woman's happiness primarily comes from the oxytocin-producing events of nurturing and being nurtured, while a man's happiness comes primarily from the testosterone-producing event of making a difference in his partner's life. Not being a man, and not being dependent on 30 times more testosterone to feel good, a woman just doesn't know what it's like.

Understanding why a man bonds so deeply with his dog may provide some useful insight to a woman, but before pursuing this analogy, let me first make a qualifying statement. Certainly a woman is not expected to behave like a pet. But there are elements of this relationship that can illuminate the nature of men and their affections.

A dog is always happy to see his owner, right? A man may have had a frustrating day at work, but when he arrives home his dog is wagging his tail and leaping with joy. His hero is home, and the dog's enthusiastic reception leaves a man feeling victorious. His testosterone level rises. His stress melts away.

> A man's desire to please a woman is much greater than her desire to please him.

This example of unconditional love and abundant appreciation from dog to man is an important indicator of the way to a man's heart. He needs to feel appreciated.

Women tend to overlook or underestimate how important it is to her man that she be delighted with him. That's because, while a man's deepest desire is to make his partner happy, hers is to find a partner who can make her happy. He wants to enchant; she wants to be enchanted. A man doesn't spend his life looking for someone to love him, as a woman does. Instead he looks for someone he can be successful in loving. Certainly a man loves to receive a woman's love, but more important for him is to feel successful in giving love.

Something else that is undervalued by women is a man's desire to protect and provide for his partner and family. Too many women take these efforts for granted. When a man struggles to make a better life for his family, a woman can easily think he's doing it for himself. She doesn't recognize that, in his heart of hearts, he does it to please her. Here's the truth: Long before she came into his life, he was preparing to provide for her and seek pleasure for her. He didn't know her name, but he knew that one day that he would find his someone to care for.

While women hope one day to find their knight in shining armor, a man's life depends on becoming that knight. Although men have difficulty expressing these feelings, they are there deep inside. Next time you listen to the radio, listen to the love songs. They are almost all written by men.

On Venus the story is different. When a woman comes home from a stressful day at work, her husband's pleasure at seeing her doesn't necessarily make her happy. She may be glad that he's happy, but his happiness doesn't lower her stress levels. If she had a particularly difficult day, it can even make her irritable to see him in such a good mood.

I can remember many times when my coming home from a trip feeling great would compel my wife to let me know how difficult things had been for her while I was away. My good mood evaporated as I heard about the disasters that occurred in my absence. My pleasure at being home did nothing to make her feel better. Instead, my happy-go-lucky attitude would prompt her to say, "You have no idea how much I do around here!"

> When a woman is unhappy, a man's happiness can actually make her more stressed.

She was certainly stating the truth, and all she was doing was giving in to her need to talk to release the stress of having to manage everything without my help. But the point I'm making is that my happiness did little to improve her mood. It did nothing to release her stress. While a man experiences testosterone-related stress relief when the woman in his life is happy, it's not so for a woman.

This isn't meant to imply that a woman is more selfish than a man, or that women don't care about men. It just means that a man's happiness is not as significant to her as hers is to him. This isn't a criticism. It's simply an important hormonal difference in the ways the genders cope with stress.

Of course, all this talk about the joy that men feel in pleasing their women leaves most women thinking, "If he wants to please me so much, why isn't he more willing to do things to help me?" It's a simple answer, really. He wants his woman to be happy but he also needs to rest at the end of the day. He can't help it—he's hard-wired that way.

Giving: A Gift for Men, a Trap for Women

One of the biggest bones of contention in any relationship is score-keeping. Who's doing the most? Who should be giving more? Nine times out of 10, it's the woman who's giving more, and while she's not happy about it, she can't seem to stop herself.

When a woman is in love, she is generally happy to do things for a man without any expectation that he give back more. This is because she's already getting what she needs. This tendency goes away, however, when she's under stress.

When a woman is stressed, instead of taking more time to get what she needs, she mistakenly gives more of herself. Just as a man needs to rest and recover after a day of action and challenge, a woman needs to balance her nonstop tendency to give by taking time during her day to also receive the support she needs. Giving of herself only stimulates maximum oxytocin when she feels she's also getting the support she needs.

> Even when a woman isn't getting what she needs, she feels the urge to give more.

Indeed, the more supported a woman feels, the more benefit she gets through unconditional giving. With increased oxytocin she is able to fully appreciate the support she has. Giving is embedded in the female psyche. Even when she isn't getting what she needs, her brain simply *remembers* that giving more makes oxytocin, and just this knowledge can make her feel better. On this basis she can continue to give and give, and yet keep her stress levels down.

While this is a perfect cycle for increasing fulfillment, it can also become a major problem. That's because, as she gives more of herself without getting her needs fulfilled, her oxytocin levels begin to drop. You would think she would stop and say, "Hey! Enough! I can't keep doing this!" But, unless she takes deliberate action to stop the cycle, she will feel a compulsive urge to give more instead of taking time to receive support and replenish her hormonal needs.

Mixed up in all of this is her plain crazy notion that *she must continue to give if she is to be deemed deserving of receiving*. Until she figures out how to put on the brakes, she'll keep running herself into the ground. Or, into the cave. This is how role reversals are born!

Giving Less to Get More

Things are very different on Mars.

There, the thing a man wants most is for his partner to be happy. If she's happy that's one less problem he must solve! Her happiness is also something he can take credit for, and we all know how much men love to claim credit, don't we? When she's happy, it's easier for him to rebuild his testosterone levels.

But there's something else that's different on Mars, something the Venusians seem to have a hard time understanding. Believe it or not, *a man from Mars loves his woman more when she gives less and is willing to receive more*!

Of course, "giving less" comes easy for a man, but not so easy for a woman. Doing something for her own benefit can seem selfish to her, so it doesn't produce the oxytocin she needs. To make more of that stress-relieving hormone, a woman needs to learn how to feel as good about receiving as she does about giving. If she clearly recognizes that she needs to receive in order to keep giving more, it can help change her perspective. Figuring out how to say "no" to the needs of the world is just as important as being able to say "yes," after all. It's just harder. But sometimes it's a bit easier for her if she tells herself that she's not saying "no" to others, but rather saying "yes" to herself. By receiving more, she'll then be able to truly give from her heart without any strings attached.

Women fear they won't be loved if they take time for themselves.

One common fear a woman may have is that if she stops giving in order to take time for herself, her man won't love her. Forget it; it's not true. A man will always love a woman more when she's getting what she needs. When a woman truly realizes this, she can release the added burden of trying to make a man happy. *By giving less she will actually get more.*

You have to understand: Men don't like feeling in debt to their women. If he owes her things, especially love, then to him their relationship is a business deal and all the romance is gone. A man's romantic love is not an obligation but a yearning in his heart. He gives it freely, not because he's obligated. Any and all expectations that he should give more to her because she has given so much to him will literally drain a man of his romantic energies and motivations.

To bring out the best in a man, simply cut him some slack.

Here's another caution, and it brings us right back to the issue of role reversal at the beginning of this chapter: Any woman who wants to bring her man back to Mars, or keep him there, must take care not to emasculate him, or, in hormonal terms, deprive him of his testosterone supply. Don't harangue a man with what he didn't do, never does do and really should do. Don't offer unsolicited advice or point out how he could have done something better. When you do that, you're giving him the message that you can do it better; that you can, in fact, do it all. So why should he bother trying? A man will react to his woman's increased masculinity with increased passivity. And that's when Mars catches fire and turns Venus to ice.

The take-away message is this: Women have the power to bring out the best in a man simply by cutting him some slack. Don't give him advice he doesn't want or need. And don't complain about what he fails to do. When a woman is undemanding, it gives him the clear message that he is doing his job—which is to make her happy. He'll feel entitled to go into his cave, but he'll come out much sooner than if she were hounding him to do something.

No surprises here; everyone knows that communication is a complicated issue. In this arena, every relationship is a work in progress. You need only to refer back to the beginning of this chapter to see how high the stakes are. Too little talk, too much talk, the wrong kind of talk—they're all communication habits so flawed that they can be role-reversing. It's difficult for any couple to figure out how to keep the love conversation going and the feel-good hormones flowing without running afoul of the gender-specific tendencies of one or the other. Men want to negotiate, if they choose to talk at all. Women err on the side of complaint. The only thing certain, though often easy to forget, is that both men and women are aiming for the same goal: happiness.

However, there's a strategy for honoring the differences between men and women while also ensuring that communication gives each of them what they want and need. It's a technique I call Venus Talk, and, come to think of it, I can't do it justice in just a few paragraphs. It deserves a chapter of its own! So, meet me in Chapter Six for more.

CHAPTER 6

WHY VENUS STOPS TALKING AND MARS STOPS LISTENING

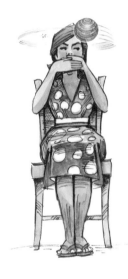
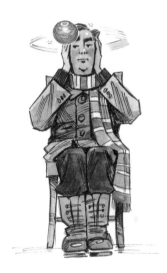

VENUS KNOWS SHE NEEDS TO TALK,
BUT SHE DOESN'T QUITE KNOW HOW TO
GET STARTED. MARS WANTS TO LISTEN, BUT
IT MAKES HIM UNCOMFORTABLE.

She says, "Why should I bother talking when he doesn't listen." *He says,* "When she gets talking, it can go on and on... then no matter what I say, it's always the wrong thing."

Many a shared household is plagued by the static of poor communication. Yes, there are problems with the transmission— bad timing, ill-chosen words, even some less-than-noble motives.

But the biggest complaint, invariably lodged by a woman, is that her man just doesn't listen.

It's true. But in defense of males everywhere, I must point out that this wasn't deemed a shortcoming until fairly recently.

In the past, men weren't expected to be good listeners. Women didn't care if a man listened, because she didn't see it as important for him to know all the details of her thoughts and feelings. For her, having a man listen only became important when her lifestyle began separating her from the community of women with whom she shared her feelings. Now that women-only gatherings are a relative rarity, there's a feeling among many busy females that something is missing in their lives, something important.

Women need to talk. When a woman doesn't get a chance to talk about her feelings throughout the day, she becomes stressed and feels an urgent need to share her feelings with her partner at home. If this need isn't met, then whatever else her man does for her is filtered by a growing belief that she isn't getting enough loving recognition. When couples don't talk and men don't listen, nothing he does for her will feel good enough.

Is it really that important? Yes, it is. Next to romance, the second biggest super-oxytocin producer in a relationship is communication. When women feel free to talk about the stresses of their day, the action creates a flood of feel-good oxytocin, the kind that restores their ability to give and nurture. But, while talking has always been a key stress reducer on Venus, many women today are actually too stressed to even sense this need. A woman may feel there's no time to talk because she has too many things to do. While this sounds plausible, the real reason she feels so harried is that she hasn't yet experienced what it's like to truly share how her days affect her, and afterward, to feel assured of having been heard.

But the possible benefits to a woman are greater than simply being heard. And, she stands to gain more than just having her stress levels reduced by talking. When a couple develops a talking routine and the woman can rely on her husband not just hearing her but truly listening, then something more powerful occurs. The woman comes to know and anticipate that there will always be someone waiting for her who not only cares about her, but also understands the challenges she faces day after day. Even while she's at work, in a testosterone-stimulating environment, just knowing that someone at home loves her and knows what she's going through can become a reliable producer of super-oxytocin for her.

But all of that is a dream for many women. She knows she needs to talk about her feelings, but she doesn't quite know how to get started. He wants to listen, but it makes him uncomfortable. The good news for women is that the problem really isn't hers to solve—at least not initially. It's the man who's in the best position to help the couple find a winning solution. But that solution doesn't look like what either of them might imagine.

For one thing, we know that this won't be the type of sharing that women engage in when they communicate, because a man is not a woman, and he's not wired to be part of a feelings-sharing session. It makes him squirm to listen to his woman's frustrations, because it's his natural tendency to want to jump in and fix the problem with a glib solution. And, to share his own feelings? Please. He'd rather have a root canal.

But I'm here to tell you that woman-to-man communication and sharing can indeed happen, because I've seen it again and again. Women find that it's actually even more stress-reducing than sharing with another woman—and, wonder of wonders, the men grow to like it and actually look forward to it.

To achieve this feat of inter-gender communication, women must learn how to share their feelings in ways their men can work with. They have to recognize their own need to share and learn to respect boundaries on their sharing. Men, meanwhile, must learn how to listen. By that I don't mean he should merely sit still and let her words wash over him mindlessly—though that's sometimes where we start! I mean real listening, the kind in which a man is actively, caringly absorbing what his woman has to say.

Over the course of my early career, I grew to recognize that couples weren't going to adopt this sort of enhanced communication practice without some sort of structure to assist them, so I began developing a model. I've used it successfully for 25 years now, and I call it **Venus Talk**. Here's how it works, in basic terms: She talks for a few minutes each day, just updating her life, always taking care not to talk about the relationship or seek solutions from her man. This goes on for 10 minutes, tops. When she's done, she thanks him for listening, because that's absolutely all the man does. He just *listens*.

I find that men readily agree to participate in a Venus Talk a couple of times a week, because it's short and simple and, most important, it doesn't require anything of him but listening. He doesn't need to talk about his feelings, or respond to her complaints, or justify himself in any way. He knows that his woman simply wants to talk to him because it makes her feel better. Hey, if it makes her happy, it makes him happy, too, men tell me.

A man can find it easier to listen when his wife respects his boundaries during their conversation.

Later in this chapter I'll provide you a detailed structure for trying your hand at my Venus Talk strategy. But first, let's back up and make sure we really understand the role this communication technique can play in modern-day relationships that are besieged by too many commitments and rocked by changes in gender roles.

What Happens When We Don't Talk

In the work world, we keep our feelings on the back burner. It's not appropriate to moan or rant with a customer or client. That's true for men on the job and for women. Everybody's there for one purpose, and that's to get the job done.

But at home and in relationships, it's a different matter. By the time women get home they're starved for some good ol' oxytocin-producing experiences. If women are to spend their days at work or isolated in their homes, they need to balance this increased testosterone born of excess responsibility with similar increases in oxytocin. Talking about the problems in her life can be a major oxytocin stimulator for a woman. But we have to remember that it's also a major testosterone depressor for him. His preferred method for reducing stress and replenishing his testosterone levels, remember, is to retreat to the cave.

So, what happens? Especially if the woman hasn't fully recognized her need to talk, but even if she has, accidents of timing and content occur. Maybe she unknowingly sabotages an otherwise pleasant moment by talking about her feelings when he finds it inappropriate to do so. Maybe she meets his request that she pick up dry cleaning with a litany of what's gone wrong in life instead of just answering, "I can't, I'm too busy." If she feels she's having a hard time getting through to him, she may consciously or unconsciously start arguments, just to get her feelings out. Or maybe it's a fine time for her to talk, but he feels she goes on for far too long. As I've mentioned in a previous chapter, the poisoned date-night conversation is a classic: She talks about how bad the food is, mostly because she wants and needs to talk about *something* to relieve her stress. But it leaves her date feeling he's failed to make her happy. And we know how important it is for a man to make his woman happy.

> When she shares her feelings at a time he feels is inappropriate, the friction can lead to an argument.

All of these are examples of how women misguidedly try to stimulate the production of oxytocin through talking that is ineffective at best and destructive at worst. On the following page is a table that shows the full range of ways that women can fail at talking—and how their men respond:

When a woman chooses to talk…	How a man feels in reaction to her timing…
When she's overwhelmed she'll wait until he asks her to do something, and then she'll enumerate in great detail everything on her to-do list as evidence that she's already doing too much.	He may feel as if he's wrong for asking for help. He feels burdened by her problems as if in some way he's let her down and her problems are his fault.
When she feels there's not enough romance in their relationship, she may wait until he wants sex to bring it up.	He may feel rejected as if she's not interested in having sex with him, or he may feel mad that she's withholding sex to get what she wants.
When she disapproves of his parenting style she may wait to bring it up until the children aren't cooperating, happy or doing well.	He may feel blamed and criticized at a time when he's most vulnerable. He feels she's being unsupportive and unappreciative of his efforts to be a good parent.
When she feels concerned about money she might wait until he's considering a purchase to bring up her issues.	He may feel controlled, as if she's suggesting that she's in charge of his spending. He misinterprets her general concern as an immediate concern about the particular purchase he's considering.
When she's upset that he's not doing what he promised she'll wait until he's engaged in some relaxing or entertaining activity like reading a book or watching TV.	He may feel annoyed that she waits until he's taking his needed recovery time and then expects him to stop and respond to her needs. He wants to respond, but feels he needs his rest.
When she wants to spend more time with him she'll wait to bring it up until he wants to spend time with a friend.	He may feel manipulated by her feelings. When he wants to take care of his own needs, suddenly she becomes needy. He cares about her feelings, but he can't do what he wants and meet her needs, too.

If you review the above list, it may seem like she's just waiting to reject, criticize, and complain, or even to control or punish him—especially if you're a man who's reading it! After a closer look, though, you begin to realize what's obvious to any woman living with a man. She has very few opportunities to share her feelings, she never knows when such an opportunity will crop up or how long it will last, and she's probably guilty only of being clumsy in how she raises the topics. She certainly doesn't wake up each morning plotting how to ruin his day. She just wants to talk more. She's hard-wired for it, with more neural connections available to her to recognize and describe feelings than he'll ever have. And she craves the hormones that talking produces.

> Women often feel there are not many opportunities to talk in a relationship.

The way to take the tension out of the interaction is to provide regular opportunities for the woman to talk and the man to listen. Knowing that she'll have the opportunity to address these matters takes away a woman's need to force the issue.

Creating Time to Talk

To a man, the scariest four words in the English language are, "We need to talk." When a woman initiates a conversation, it puts the man on the defensive. He feels as though she's asking him to do something he can't do. Not surprisingly, then, woman-initiated talks don't get very far. She finds he doesn't have much to say. But when it's the man making the appointment, it works much better. If he understands that talking would make her happy, and that the conversation isn't going to pull him out of his comfort zone, he's usually more than willing to comply.

What exactly is his comfort zone? Not talking, basically. If "talking" means that she talks and he simply listens to support her in feeling better, he can agree to that. However, if it means he's going to be expected to talk about his feelings, the deal's off. Even more distasteful to him would be a situation in which she's going to talk about her feelings and then ask him to participate with her in solving day-to-day relationship-based problems. Mixing emotions with problem solving is all but illegal on Mars; sorry, no can do.

This is frustrating to Venusians. They're all about mixing emotions with problem solving—it's practically the planetary pastime! But if women want to talk about their feelings and get some oxytocin made in the process, they must be willing to meet their men on his gender-specific terms and give up the problem solving part of it. Take it to a girlfriend instead, ladies. Your man is going to meet you half way, but he'll go no further. He's not moving to Venus.

And women should be glad of this! As we've already seen, when a woman actually does succeed in motivating her man to be more like a woman, she loses her attraction for him. It weakens him, and it may even result in the role reversal that sets Mars afire and Venus on ice. I'm not saying a man can't have a well-developed sensitive side. I'm saying they must retain a strong masculine side.

Women who are loving and compassionate—and smart—will accede to a man's wish to keep daily issues and thorns in the relationship separate from getting her feelings heard. In so doing, she's keeping the talking task something her man can agree to. He'll see it as *his* version of problem solving—getting her feelings heard—and that way of looking at it will elevate his testosterone levels and reduce his stress.

> During a Venus Talk, she shares her feelings and he just listens.

Ladies, the only place you can get your feelings heard *and* your problems solved by a man is in the therapist's office. That's the insight you need to hang onto. Women who insist upon mixing emotions with problem solving find their men become restless, irritable and then depressed. He may begin to interrupt and offer solutions that she doesn't want to hear. As a result, she feels more stress instead of less. His testosterone levels drop almost visibly. To prevent things from escalating into a fight, women need to give their men the ability to not respond at all. And men need to learn the art of listening without interrupting to impose a solution.

The final boundary that must not be crossed in a conversation designed to get a women's feelings heard pertains to content. A woman doesn't get free rein to say whatever she wants, no matter how hurtful, while a man sits passively and listens. To do so would be unfair, but moreover, it wouldn't serve her needs. As long as she's in a problem solving mode and trying to fix him, she's making testosterone, not stress-releasing oxytocin.

Enough of my talk for now; let's get *you* talking!

Initiating a Venus Talk

The secret to a successful Venus Talk begins with scheduling. Get it on the calendar or the Blackberry—don't wait until the woman is so stressed and oxytocin-starved that she demands attention. That will result in her doing all the don'ts I've been talking about. Plus, she won't achieve the hormone-producing results she seeks. Just the pressure of "having to get something out" can restrict the production of this stress-reducing hormone. So, plan your Venus Talk much as you would a date.

Venus Talks are much more effective when they're planned

A Venus Talk should last about 10 minutes and should be practiced at least three times a week. During each session the woman needs only to express how she feels about the challenges in her life, and the man needs only to listen and occasionally murmur encouragement or ask a question. He isn't allowed to make comments, and she's not allowed to ask for them. But if she falls silent, he can be helpful by encouraging her to "tell me more."

When the 10 minutes are up, the woman should thank her man for his time and attention and he should respond by giving her a big hug. Talking about the Venus Talk should then be off-limits to both parties for at least 12 hours. Both man and woman need a chance to savor the interaction. For her, it was stress relief, and it felt great! For him, it was the pleasure of having pleased her, and that doesn't feel bad either.

For those of you who are want more guidance on what should transpire during a 10-minute Venus Talk, read on.

Using the Venus Talking Points

The Venus Talking Points outlined below are a simple guide to how you can proceed, especially when this communication discipline is a new one for you. They consist of six questions a man can ask his woman to get her talking and keep her talking, which is the goal here, for sure! She can answer by talking about her day, her week, her past, her childhood or simply whatever comes into her mind. The right answer is whatever comes into her heart and mind.

The Venus Talking Points

1. What makes you feel frustrated?
2. What makes you feel disappointed?
3. What makes you feel concerned?
4. What makes you feel embarrassed?
5. What do you wish, want or need?
6. What do you appreciate, understand or trust?

Take about 90 seconds for each question, allowing the woman to answer by sharing whatever comes to her mind—it may be one topic or many. Our subconscious mind knows what's bothering us, and it will automatically release our stress when given an opportunity. All we need is to ask the questions and share what comes up. Taking a brief time to explore and share whatever comes to mind in response to each question causes oxytocin levels to rise.

While answering the first five questions, it's best to steer clear of letting the woman talk about her partner, but with the last question I recommend that the answers be addressed directly to him—expressing feelings of gratitude and appreciation. For him, the appreciation will come as a great reward for the time and effort he has invested. It will also stimulate his testosterone levels, because he has been successful in making her happy.

Why do we limit these Venus Talks to 10 minutes? There's a good reason. We're training the mind and body to release stress in a shorter period of time. It also helps to release the man from the testosterone-oriented trap of always setting and achieving goals. By saying from the outset that 10 minutes is the limit, he is prevented from even thinking about how long it should go.

In the beginning, because this is new, a Venus Talk may feel mechanical, and the questions I've provided may seem rote or arbitrary. The woman may have difficulty talking for the entire 10 minutes, though perhaps the time will seem too short. Regardless, the pair should stick to the time limit and gradually they'll become more patient with the structure. Over a few sessions, the woman will train her mind and body to begin producing more oxytocin within a shorter and shorter period of time, gaining the maximum benefit for her body's stress relief.

Keep in mind that the Venus Talk structure doesn't lock you in. At other times in your life you can certainly have other kinds of conversations. What you'll find is that regularly-scheduled Venus Talks will make other conversations much more stress-free. It's said that money is the number one reason couples fight. But underlying any topic of contention is stress. People who argue are stressed. But, thanks to the Venus Talks technique, both women and men benefit from increased release of stress-reducing hormones. Just as her oxytocin levels go up when she talks about her feelings, his testosterone levels go up when he feels he's making a positive difference in her life.

This kind of one-sided conversation is unusual. It's certainly not the way women talk to one another on Venus. But it's probably as close as a man can get to understanding his woman without becoming one! When women talk they will naturally mix feelings with a gradual tendency to move toward problem solving. The empathy they show one another helps release stress so they can have a better perspective with which to eventually solve a problem. The same can be true of couples that practice Venus Talk strategy, if they're willing to stick with it and believe in it.

I once counseled a woman who greatly resisted the Venus Talk process. It seemed so artificial and insincere, she said. She didn't want to talk with someone who wasn't interested in what she had to say, she told me. That was her big complaint, and it was true. Her husband wasn't at all interested in what she talked about. But once she tried Venus Talk, she was amazed by how good she felt. She knew her partner was not particularly interested in her topics, but she had never been able to talk about anything without him interrupting before. That alone made it rewarding for her. Eventually, as he got better at listening to her in Venus Talk, he became interested in almost everything she said. All of their communication improved, and soon even relationship topics weren't off-limits.

Venus Talks can indeed open doors that have long been closed between men and women. But it doesn't happen overnight, nor should it. For the first year of Venus Talks, it's important that the woman not address any problems she has with her man. If she were to do so, it would only make it harder for him to hear what she's saying, and for her to feel heard. But in time it will become easier for him to hear her complaints and deal with them without taking them personally.

Let's look at some questions that may arise when couples institute Venus Talks:

What if the man dislikes being only the listener?

Some men need to feel successful at something before they get really interested in doing it. So, praise him early and often! Once he discovers that he can make his woman happy by listening, he'll find it worthwhile to stay involved.

What if he interrupts or tries to offer solutions?

At the beginning of each Venus Talk the woman needs to remind her man that he should simply listen without trying to solve things for her. By reminding him that he doesn't have to say anything or fix anything she's also reminding herself that she's not expecting him to do anything. Venus Talks can work only if she has no expectations for him to do anything.

What if the woman's main daily challenge is how little her man helps her, and it's really difficult for her to avoid mentioning it during the Venus Talk?

Complaining isn't the answer. If the woman shares how much she has to do, he may get the message and try to help out more. She should focus on releasing her stress. I've found that the less the woman hopes or wishes that he'd step up more, the better she'll feel—and the more he may eventually choose to do.

What if the woman begins to complain during the Venus Talk, or the man gets frustrated or angered by something she's said?

You may need a time-out to avoid an argument. Sometimes it helps for one party to write an email to the other—not to pick up the dispute, but to suggest how the next Venus Talk could end better.

What if the man continues to try to problem-solve? Or, what if relationship issues or domestic problems creep into the Venus Talk?

Maybe it's time for a **Mars Meeting**. Such sessions are all about problem solving, and they're the opposite of a Venus Talk. In a Mars Meeting the woman is the one who holds back. She doesn't share her feelings. Instead she conveys in as few words as possible the problem at hand. Since this is usually an impossible task for a woman who is under stress, it's extremely important for couples to have Venus Talks before attempting a Mars Meeting. After achieving stress release for both parties in a Venus Talk, it's usually easy for the couple to share what isn't working and what ought to be done about it.

What about men? Don't they deserve their own forum for talking about feelings?

Certainly men like to share feelings, but only in certain special circumstances—like after making love or while watching the moon rise with the woman they love. Remember, Venus Talks are about releasing stress, and men don't release stress by talking about feelings. Besides, it's not good for a man to rely on his woman as his sounding board. Remember Chapter Five and the problem of role reversal! We must also bear in mind that men are not women. When a man cares for the feelings of his woman, his romantic attraction to her grows. But when a woman cares for her man's feelings, she may become more maternal. She tends to move over to her testosterone-producing male side and take too much responsibility for him. This not only weakens him but adds an additional burden of stress to her large and growing load.

What if a couple tries Venus Talk and really dislikes it, or there's one of them who finds it pointless?

I would suggest using the *Venus Talking Points* first of all, and then that you commit yourself to at least three Venus Talks before deciding if it's worth your time. It has proved to be immensely helpful for millions of people. I've written about and taught this technique in a variety of ways for more than 25 years.

Why Venus Talks Work

Have you ever had the experience of asking for a back scratch, only to find you can't pinpoint exactly where the itch is? "A little to the left, no right, up, left again, yeah, yeah that's it, oh thank youuuu." Venus Talks are a little like that. You can't be sure where you're going or where you'll end up, and you can't expect starbursts. But you get them sometimes, and then it's great!

As we've seen, this form of non-goal-oriented communication:

- Raises levels of anti-stress hormones for both men and women

- Helps women identify and name their feelings

- Helps men learn to listen with interest, and more importantly, without interrupting or jumping to conclusions or solutions

- Frees men from the omnipresent feeling that they ought to fix something

- Gives men a deeper understanding of who their women are and what problems they face

- Helps couples avoid arguments by offering a non-confrontational forum for airing issues

- Encourages empathy in men and appreciation in women

- Helps men who are going through a difficult time to focus on their women's problems and forget their own

- Enables men, over time, to become more comfortable with communication and more forthcoming in conversations that aren't part of the Venus Talk structure

- Prompts men to begin including their women in their thinking and decision-making processes

Whew, that's a lot of benefit in a short list! I may be in danger of overselling it, but to me the Venus Talk technique offers something akin to a peace treaty in the ongoing War of the Sexes. Try it and stick with it, and I believe you'll achieve new levels of mutual satisfaction in your relationship.

Regular communication that respects gender differences does more than reduce stress, after all. It also stimulates the hormones of love and desire. We should all be working toward ever-greater understanding of the ways that men are men and women are women, hormones and all, because it's in our differing strengths and weaknesses that we will find the balance and richness that makes love last and grow.

In that spirit of mutual understanding, we will use the next chapter to home in on one of the essential traits of being a man—the tendency we have to withhold action until we can foresee nothing but trouble from waiting any longer. So, turn the page with me and meet... Emergency Man!

CHAPTER 7

EMERGENCY MAN— THE REAL REASON WOMEN NEED YOU

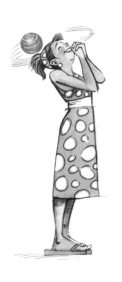
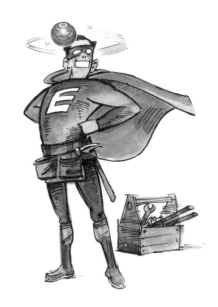

MARS COMES ALIVE IN TESTOSTERONE-STIMULATING SITUATIONS—PROJECTS THAT ANYBODY BUT EMERGENCY MAN WOULD GIVE UP ON.

Suppose I told you, a woman, that all the jobs in the household are yours. The man of the house won't have any regular chores or expectations, because you're going to do it all. Would you say, "Okay, fine, can do," or would you beg to differ? Or... might you say, "That's the deal I've got right now, so what's the difference?"

I think many women would put themselves in the third category. The men in their lives basically don't punch in for work around the house unless they are direly, desperately, catastrophically needed.

In this chapter I'm going to show these women how they can change nothing and still change absolutely everything about who does what at home. All they have to do is picture their man as a superhero named... Emergency Man!

Emergency Man (or Mr. Oblivious, as some women may also know him) is chronically unable to see dirt, clutter, full wastebaskets, dirty dishes, broken hinges, snowy driveways, clogged gutters—well, you get the picture, even if he doesn't. His visual acuity is just about nil after 5 p.m. each day. But show him an emergency and he fairly leaps into action! He swashbuckles his way through every critical situation his woman sets before him. The difference between what he won't do and what he will is measured not in how hard it is to do, or how long it takes, but by the urgency in his woman's eyes. When he knows that no one else can step up to the task, that's when Emergency Man steps in.

If you have an Emergency Man in your house, this chapter is for you. If you are Emergency Man, please skip ahead a few pages to the next topic.

How to Summon Emergency Man

Today's women need more help than they're getting. With many of them working outside the home, either they work almost another full day after rush hour or they find some help. But, whether or not you can afford a nanny or a house-cleaner, there are still tasks upon tasks upon tasks that need doing. Bills to be paid. Kids to be shuttled. Seasonal work in the yard. Recycling. Garage cleaning. The list goes on and on.

When I was growing up, my mother did virtually everything at home and at least seemed content. But she had the time to do it. Today's women do not. Even with their expanded role in the workplace, the housework remains largely theirs. Is there a way out of the situation? Probably not. But, by making some adjustments in her approach, a typical woman can get more help from her man. She just has to do a little strategizing. She has to figure out what motivates him to want to help and feel able to help.

Enter Emergency Man. Unlike a woman, Emergency Man is not the sort to feel motivated toward oxytocin-producing activities like cooking, cleaning, and taking care of the kids. No, Emergency Man craves the thrill of victory and thrives on brinksmanship. His goal in life is to be the guy who steps in just in time to save the day. And for whom does he do it? His loving woman, who looks on adoringly and applauds his every triumph over the leaky faucet, the tricky lawnmower or the boxes piled in the hallway.

Men come alive in testosterone-stimulating situations. Forget the routine; he wants the emergencies, the difficult projects, and the head-scratching problems that anybody but Emergency Man would give up on.

So give him an emergency, ladies. Don't fight his nature; make every job an assault on Mount Everest. Believe it or not, he'll thank you for it.

Women will get more support in the home when they stop expecting men to be like them—creatures who work continually for the good of the household. If a man knows he can come home from his job and retreat to the cave, catching no flack from anybody, he'll rebuild the testosterone he used up during the day and through the week. And he'll be ready to take on whatever she throws at him—as long as she can make it seem really, really important.

> Since a man thrives in situations that stimulate testosterone, let him take care of emergencies.

This takes creativity. Appealing to a man's sense of responsibility to his family won't do it. As he sees it, he discharges that responsibility every day at work. He comes home tired and yearning for the comfort of the cave. He's not coming out unless there's an emergency.

Fortunately for women, these emergencies don't always have to be urgent or big. All she has to do is point out all the things that really can't be put off much longer, and make him feel that he's the only man who can remedy the situation before trouble occurs. If he's had enough time in the cave, he'll come out and get to work. Don't drum your nails or try to drag him out early. The more support he's had for going in the cave, the faster he'll come out.

What this means is what I said at the top of the chapter— today's woman needs to assume that the chores are all hers. By not expecting more of her man, she'll save herself a lot of disappointment and resentment. But I'm not advocating that she treat him like a guest. I'm saying she should picture him as Emergency Man.

Certainly there is some overlap in gender-based household roles, and there ought to be. But once we understand the hormonal realities of the differences between men and women, the insight helps us understand that there's no point in fighting it. He's the guy who should go out in a driving rain to search for the missing family dog. And she's the one who should stay home and get dinner on the table, without a moment's guilt for staying warm and dry. The testosterone released by his task makes him feel good. The oxytocin she enjoys from her nurturing task makes her feel good, too.

Does this sound old-fashioned? I think it's realistic. And it's actually a modernized version of the gender roles as they once existed. Instead of handling only the emergencies related to the feeding and protection of the family, today's man can be expected to handle "emergencies" that arise in the domestic setting as well. The advantage to women is that they can then honestly say that they don't have to handle everything.

Emergencies, then, are matters to be defined slightly differently than we might traditionally. Today's emergencies are those that arise outside the daily routine of shopping, cooking, cleaning, and caring for the kids. They are the straws that break the camel's back: the leaks in the roof, the crashed computer, the non-functioning appliances, the weather damage to the house, the injured kid, the car repairs, and the legal/financial surprises. Even the crisis of having no milk for breakfast can be a job for Emergency Man.

The implied deal is that Venus lets Mars get the cave rest he needs when he needs it, knowing that he'll replenish his testosterone supplies. That way, when she has to ask for extra support, for back-up if you will, he's not just available but willing. And the side benefit to her is his enhanced energy for romance. Emergencies, even when they're "emergencies," create lots of testosterone for men.

The deal is fair. He gets to enjoy his rest guilt free, and when she needs help, she gets to give him a project guilt free. That's providing, of course, that he always says yes to the requests, and he should. But saying yes doesn't mean he'll get up and do it on the spot. Fulfilling her requests should be according to his timetable, unless there is a true, time-sensitive emergency.

> When a man is rested, he then has the energy and time to be her Emergency Man.

How does she know it will get done? How can she avoid having to ask again and again? By posting a list of numbered priorities and gaining his agreement that if something's on the list, he's going to do it when he can get to it.

It won't work for a woman to skip the list and demand immediate compliance. If a woman doesn't respect a man's need to prioritize and be in charge of his actions, he will eventually resist her requests. He needs to feel in charge of himself and his time if he's going to be expected to take on more duties.

So, everybody has rights. She has the right to ask and keep asking while he has the right to postpone until he is ready. To make this process more graceful, when he wants to postpone doing something, he can simply say, "Put it on the list." If that starts happening too often, she can simply say, "Honey, there are about 10 things on the list now, so when you get time, would you cross a few off?" Don't worry; he won't balk. By the time 10 things build up on the list it, that looks enough like an emergency to stimulate his brain to release some testosterone. That will give him the energy and motivation to get it done.

You should know that the emergency center in a man's brain (the amygdala) is twice as big as a woman's and only gets activated when the man perceives an urgent situation requiring his action. This center activates his emotional responses and triggers dopamine production to motivate him toward a solution. Women generally can't relate to this, because their emergency center is firing all the time about the various things that need her attention. This is because women are designed to care for children. Meanwhile, if a man is built primarily to stand guard against dangers that might threaten the people he loves, he can't have an amygdala that fires as frequently as hers. He must stay focused and calm to handle the big emergencies. That could be fire, flood or just a 10-item to-do list.

> Creating a list of household priorities helps feed a man's need to be in charge.

That list is key. It allows men to set their own schedule. It frees a woman from having to nag. As long as men hold up their end and perform their tasks within a reasonably expected period of time, women get the support they need. And that's a super-oxytocin producer for her, just knowing that his support is always available.

He Needs Space, She Needs Time

When couples have complaints about one another, it usually involves some behavior or tendency that he or she doesn't understand. Having a grasp of the differences between men and women at the hormonal level is a huge boost to any loving relationship. We grow in our ability to accept our partners as they are, without resistance, resentment or rejection. Acceptance is the foundation on which Emergency Man performs best. So it's worth our while to take some time to think about one of the more frustrating differences between men and women: that men need space to be alone in a relationship and women need time to be together.

When a woman complains about a man's cave time or his need for space, she's forgetting what a major testosterone producer his self-isolation is for him. She doesn't relate, because to her, time alone is only good for one thing: getting a break from all the giving they do. Women lessen stress by connecting with their partners, not pulling away. Talking and sharing is generally how women rebuild their stress-reducing hormones. There is one exception, though, and that's when women use alone time to do things that nurture themselves. That will produce oxytocin and provide stress relief. But, unfortunately, not many women manage to do this. Just the thought of it can be overwhelming for some women. They feel, "There's no time for me—I have too much to do."

This difference can't be solved. It must be accepted.

I guess we could say that for these women, the thought of stopping to smell the roses brings up only fears of thorns. For such women, it doesn't work to have their men say, "Quit worrying and just get away from it for a while, enjoy yourself." Such a comment is a problem solver, and it will produce testosterone for the man who says it. But it won't make any oxytocin for the woman who hears it. Want to know what does? A different sort of comment: "Honey, you do so much for so many people. Let me give you a hug." Now that's a comment that helps. That kind of oxytocin support helps her take a deep breath and get her bearings again.

> Just the thought of taking time for herself can feel overwhelming for some women.

Of course, as we've seen in other chapters, there are more and more women in testosterone-stimulating jobs. Such women will be drawn to the cave, just as their men are. Testosterone-stimulating jobs inevitably deplete this hormone for women just as they would for men, and some form of cave time is required for replenishment. But, no matter how much a woman thinks she needs to retreat to the cave, her man will always need it far more. A man's need to rebuild testosterone ranges from 10 to 30 times greater than a woman's, just because men use so much more of it.

If women have difficulty taking time for themselves to recover from stress, the equivalent difficulty for men is being there for others. Women enjoy gathering in a cooperative or collaborative manner at the end of the day. Invite a man, however, and all you'll do is drain the little energy he has left. Just as his cave time does little for her, her desire to share and spend time together does virtually nothing to help him cope with stress.

After a very testosterone-oriented day, a woman needs more than to rebuild her testosterone levels, though. She also needs to boost her oxytocin levels. Testosterone-rebuilding may get her ready for the next day, but she will continue to be stressed until she's made sufficient oxytocin. Unreleased stress not only prevents her from getting in touch with her positive feelings, it interferes with her health as well. I have repeatedly observed women having fertility issues because they aren't effectively coping with the stress of their testosterone-stimulating jobs. These women often cope with the stress of work by being alone for a time or through solitary exercise, but these won't help her transition back to her female side. She needs oxytocin. Many women have restored their fertility by increasing their access to oxytocin-stimulating behaviors, therapies, and foods.

Our Communication Styles Often Clash

Now let's work our way back to Emergency Man and look at how women should handle his care and feeding. Communication and stress relief may not seem like essential elements, but they are.

Men are naturally motivated to communicate in ways that will lower stress in men. They have no idea that this same style of communicating may increase a woman's stress levels. To release his stress, a man tends to either solve the problem or dismiss it in some way. To release her stress, a woman is looking for a warmer, more supportive response. This is a Mars-Venus collision in the making. He thinks he is simply being helpful when he expresses an opinion, but she feels he's either being cold and heartless or he must not understand what she's saying.

Here are some examples of men sounding dismissive:

"Don't worry about it."

"Here's what you should do..."

"Just let it go."

"It's not that important."

"That's not what happened."

"That's not what he means."

"You're expecting too much."

"That's just the way things are.

"Don't get so upset."

"You shouldn't let them talk to you that way."

"Do whatever you want."

"Don't let them get to you like that."

"It's simple, just say…"

"All you have to do is…"

"Forget it."

"It's not such a big deal."

"Look! There's nothing more you can do about it!"

"You shouldn't feel that way."

On Mars these short comments are intended to be supportive, but on Venus they can be insulting. Maybe if she's in problem-solving mode they can be helpful, but if she's upset they will sound anything but. They may even seem condescending. In short, these are testosterone-producing statements, not oxytocin-producing. They give her the message to not bother him unless she has a real emergency. This certainly is not a very good invitation for her to ask for his help when she needs it.

Instead of stepping in with a fix-it comment, a man is more stress-relieving to a woman by listening, making reassuring or sympathetic sounds, and asking questions. And of course he can use the Venus Talk technique described in Chapter Six, which requires him to say nothing more than "Tell me more." It's his staying power as well as his attention and focus on what she's saying and feeling that will increase her oxytocin levels.

Men can enhance communication with their partners by listening more instead of jumping in with a quick-fix solution.

Giving solutions or minimizing the problem tends to increase testosterone and lower her oxytocin levels.

In these ways and others, without knowing it or intending it, a man can give his woman the message that he's not willing to be her Emergency Man. And, without bearing in mind how men think, women will deprive themselves of having an Emergency Man—just because she'll lack the courage and persistence to ask for what she wants. This is a critical issue in any couple's efforts to improve mutual understanding. As women do a better job of communicating their needs, their men will listen and learn. And soon these men will see that whether it's a capital-E Emergency or a lower case-e emergency, what their women are asking for is truly an emergency. She needs help! That's all it will take for him to find the energy to pitch in. When he does, she'll come to rely on him and trust him instead of resenting him, and that's a super-oxytocin producer if ever there was one.

The Home Improvement Committee

As is true of everything in Mars' and Venus' universe, there are as many knocks on one gender as there are on another. I hope you're ready, ladies, because here come yours!

One of the biggest mistakes a woman can make—and one that can hinder her ability to have her own Emergency Man—is to give unsolicited advice. Women love getting advice. They even expect it. Advice is a form of help, and offers of help are oxytocin-producing. They also give a woman a feeling of togetherness with the woman providing the advice or help. That's why it's tempting for a woman to think a man would like her advice, just to promote that same spirit of togetherness in their relationship. Sometimes she becomes so excited about this new opportunity that she forms what I call a home-improvement committee. Its aim is mostly to improve him! Just as men tend to have a Mr. Fix-It gene, women tend to have a Home Improvement gene that predisposes her to making her man just that much better. She thinks she's being loving, and that she's celebrating togetherness.

Well, men love doing things with their partners, especially if the doing makes her happy. But they have a greater need to do things on their own. That's why men don't immediately ask for directions or other sorts of help. So for her to offer advice is downright annoying. He may even think of it as nagging.

Here are a few examples of a woman's *Home Improvement Committee*:

"Are you going to wear that tie?"

"Have you eaten today?"

"Did you talk to your lawyer about this?"

"Why do you need to buy a new one?"

"When are you going to put this away?"

"Isn't it time for you to get a hair cut?"

"You should buy new t-shirts. These have holes."

"You should slow down, you could get a ticket."

"When are you going to clean up this office?"

"How can you think with that music so loud?"

"When are you going to cut the grass?"

"Next time we should read the reviews."

"Did you wash your hands?"

"You've already had one dessert."

"You're not giving yourself enough time to rest."

"Try planning more in advance."

"You forgot the box. Maybe if you'd put it out you'd have remembered."

"Remember to make reservations."

"Your closet needs attention."

A better way to nurture a man is to give him lots of space to do things the way he wants to do them. Rather than look for ways to change and improve him, look for things that he does right and show that you appreciate him. When a woman acknowledges what a man has done, she helps to restore his testosterone levels. Just coming home to a woman who is grateful for his support helps a man to relax and restore his energies, resulting in less time needed in the cave!

Accepting Our Natural Differences

The more aware we are of our natural differences, the more tolerant we can become of them when they arise. Instead of wondering what's wrong with our partner, we can take the nuanced step of pondering what may be wrong with our approach to them. Instead of assuming that our partner is being inconsiderate on purpose, we can just consider them clueless, or, as I said above, oblivious. That's not a put-down. It's the truth. From time to time, we just don't have a clue as to what our partners are doing or why. We're just different.

> It is comforting to remember that our partners mean well but are often clueless.

Accepting our differences immediately lightens our relationships. Many couples feel a heaviness in their lives because they believe they have to sacrifice themselves, and at least partially give up who they are to please their partners. This attitude needs to change.

Certainly every relationship requires making adjustments, compromises, and sacrifices, but it doesn't have to feel like we're giving up who we are! Instead, we can choose to see it as a compromise. Life isn't about having everything our own way. It's about sharing and sacrificing. When we realize this, we experience the true opening of our lives and the growth of our love.

Sacrifice is a negative-sounding word, but we can make it positive when we recognize that the sacrifice is worthwhile. It can be an act of love that is, like the root of the word, sacred. What was it but a sacrifice when I gave up my sleep in past decades to comfort a sick or frightened child? To me it was sacred, for it enabled my heart to grow.

But let me take the discussion down a notch now, to a level more easily related to the everyday sacrifices we make in loving relationships. If I want to drive fast and my wife wants me to slow down, I might feel that I have to sacrifice my need for speed for her need for safety. I might even feel controlled and resist a compromise. But, by understanding her need for oxytocin-producing support, the sacrifice becomes reasonable and worthwhile. Slowing down becomes less a sacrifice and more a simple adjustment or compromise, because I care about my wife's feelings and preferences. Driving fast lowers my stress levels, because as a man, any simple action followed by a desired response stimulates my testosterone production. The better the car performs, the better I feel. But I raise my wife's stress levels when I drive fast, so I don't. It's not that I have to give up driving fast; it just means that when she's riding with me, I need to drive slower. And that's just a small example of how what once could have seemed like an unreasonable request can take on new meaning once we understand the different ways men and women handle and release stress.

> When we understand our different ways of coping with stress, compromise becomes easier.

Let's now look at a few examples that pertain to women: *horseback riding and shoe shopping.*

Riding a horse can be said to have an element of risk, much like driving a car fast. However, horseback riding lowers a woman's stress levels. It's because she's in a nurturing (oxytocin-producing) relationship with the horse. She feeds and grooms the horse, and in return, the horse carries her to her destination. Horseback riding requires sensitivity, patience, and most importantly, the willingness to trust in a real partnership. Not surprisingly, more than 70 percent of all riders today are women.

For women shopping for shoes or other accessories is a super-oxytocin producer that reduces stress. Look in a woman's closet and you'll find rows of shoes in a variety of colors for every season, mood or outfit. She can tell you the season's top colors... and the list is long and full of funny names like "puce." Top colors this season for men? Same as last year and every other: Black and brown.

The variety of colors and textures seen when a woman shops is pure candy for her. It overwhelms him. She moves along looking left and right, up and down. If he's been forced to accompany her, he drags along looking straight ahead, hoping either to see a bench or an exit sign. She uses the trip as an oxytocin-building opportunity, seeking to meet the needs of others—cards for friends, toys for children, a blouse for her mother. He, however, is scraping the bottom of his testosterone supply. If he doesn't find a Radio Shack soon, he may die.

The difference here isn't that men hate shopping and women love it. It's that women shop for the fun of discovery, and men need a clear destination and goal. And, if a woman wants her man to go at it with any zeal, of course, she needs to get that goal on the list for... Emergency Man!

Our Brains are Wired Differently

You may think I've said as much as I need to say about men, women and shopping, but I do hope to leave you with an understanding of gender-based brain differences before I leave both the example and the chapter behind. It takes us right back to why women need an Emergency Man.

So indulge me: Why do women have such an affinity for shopping? Well, it could be because she has 40 percent more connective tissue between the left and right sides of the brain. While men tend to use one side at a time, women tend to use both sides no matter what they're doing.

In practical terms, this means that when a man uses his right brain—the side geared to fun—the left and more serious side will become inactive and rest. But when a woman uses the fun and creative right side of her brain, she still remains connected to the serious left. She may be doing something fun and enjoyable but another part of her brain is still aware of all her responsibilities. Do you now see why she has such needs in her life? Can you understand now, gentlemen, why so many things she wants you to do really are emergencies? Her list is long, and it's always there in front of her, no matter what else she's doing.

> Showing mutual respect for our differences will enrich our love.

The more we understand our gender-based hormonal differences, the easier it is for men and women to get along and have their needs met. Instead of expecting our partners to think and act the way we do, we are then able to consider what we could do or say that would be in their best interests. On this foundation of understanding and goodwill, we can build mutual respect and an ever-growing appreciation, if that's our goal. Can such a pursuit do anything but serve to enrich our love?

In the next chapter, we'll delve more into gender-based differences and how they play out in a relationship. We'll see how they can contribute to finding love and building a long-term relationship, but we'll also see how, if we're not careful, these differences can destroy relationships.

CHAPTER 8

VENUS AND MARS COLLIDE INTO LOVE

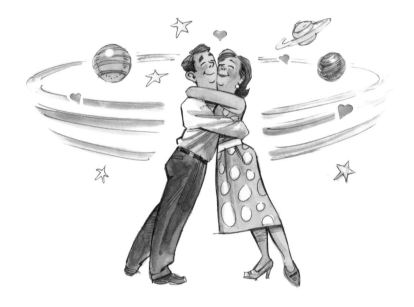

TO TRULY GIVE EQUAL RESPECT WE MUST FIRST
RECOGNIZE THAT WE ARE DIFFERENT AND
SUPPORT THOSE DIFFERENCES.

In his idealized relationship, a typical man still fantasizes of
coming home each day to a completely fulfilled partner who has
not only prepared a gourmet dinner and made a welcoming fire in
the fireplace, but strewn rose petals in the direction of the bedroom.
While most women today don't have the time or energy to help
their men live this fantasy, the average woman has her own modest
yet unrealistic dream. She wishes to have a loving and supportive

husband awaiting her when she, too, comes home from work. She doesn't need him to be holding a wire whisk or a feather duster or a long-stemmed rose. She just wants a kiss, a warm word, and the certain knowledge that he adores her. She wants a wife.

In various ways and to differing degrees, women want their men to be more like women. Now that they're working and are time-pressed, they want men to share equal responsibility at home and in the relationship. It's no longer sufficient for a man to be a good provider. If she's working outside the home as well as in it, she figures he, too, should be working inside the home as well as out. And, in her opinion, he could stand to be a little more present in the relationship, too. He should be a sympathetic partner who is eager to talk about the day's stresses and share in all routine domestic duties. When the day is done, he should put out a few of the domestic fires that crop up in any household—crooked mailbox, crumbling plaster, shorted out electrical circuit—and then whisk her away to a romantic date that he has planned in every detail.

But men have their own set of preferences. Just as wives want their husbands to change with the times, husbands want their wives to stay just as their mothers were 30 years ago or more. They believe that women should be domestic divas, yet nurturing, and attentive to every need of their men. They're oblivious, of course. They have no idea what sort of creativity and skill it takes to create a pleasant and well-functioning home.

Stress levels escalate when unrealistic expectations collide with modern realities.

Venus and Mars have had their orbits knocked off-kilter. It's a struggle for any couple today to figure out how to form and maintain a relationship, and the stresses are showing.

Much of the tension arises from the changed role of women, of course. Women today carry a burden twice that of their mothers.

They not only feel the economic pressure to work outside the home, but also an ancient and perhaps genetic imperative to work in the home. Unlike a man, a woman's nurturing instincts and nesting urges encompass a unique set of inherited wishes, wants, needs, and standards developed by a long line of capable and proud foremothers. But, unlike her own mother, today's woman tries to live out that inheritance while also earning a living and working 9 to 5.

The stress for women today is about more than just the job. I'll explain that by drawing a contrast. Most men love a beautiful and orderly home, yet they can easily come home to an untended house and simply relax while watching TV. It just doesn't matter to a guy that much. In his world, relaxing is the highest priority, so at home he really doesn't see anything but his easy chair. Indeed, after a long day at work a man takes a deep breath and begins to relax at just the thought of going home.

It is so different for women. As she begins to think of heading home, her stress levels begin to rise. She thinks of the unwashed dishes and the piles of laundry that await her. Every cell in her body says, "My house needs to be clean before I can relax." Rest? Ha! Her mind is tyrannized by the domestic standards she feels she ought to be upholding. Over the course of the day, her brain has put together a long to-do list, one that must be fully checked-off before she can put her feet up or do anything enjoyable.

> Heading home from work, men want to relax, but women feel the pressure of a never ending to-do list.

A man has his own to-do list, of course, but it's probably still on his desk at work. He's at liberty at 5 p.m., and his wife doesn't understand why he doesn't feel motivated to use some of his "free time" to share some of the responsibilities of running the home. Isn't it his home, too?

To resolve this inevitable collision of roles and responsibilities, men and women can only hope to understand one another better. Men need to recognize the burdens that weigh down their women and work to avoid pressuring her to create the perfect home. She's already under considerable pressure. Even the slightest nudge from him could push her over the edge. At the same time, women need to recognize the limits of what men can and can't do to be more supportive. He's simply not going to become a woman.

Most men are just not equipped to be the domestic/communicative/romantic partners women seem to want today. They may try to fulfill the fantasy for a while, maybe even for years. But when the wheels finally come off, it's not just the guys who are going to end up frustrated and disillusioned. Lucky is the man whose wife appreciates what he can offer her without asking him to tie himself into knots. Luckier is the female who has the sense to accept a man as he is, because she stands to get more and more from him.

Women can't live up to the sepia-toned male fantasies, either. It is unrealistic for a man to expect a woman to create a beautiful home without his help, always be in a good mood without him fulfilling any of her needs, and be romantically available at the drop of a hat. Many women try to fulfill this fantasy in pursuit of love, but end up feeling cheated and betrayed when the results don't match the plan. Lucky is the man who is able to understand a woman's needs for help around the house, good communication, and regular romantic attention, for his is a truly happy woman.

Finding Real Love

For all the fantasizing we do, the truth is that the fantasy of love is but a poor imitation of the reality we seek—a strong, supportive, fun relationship built on mutual understanding. It's real love that we want, and if we search for a partner with realistic expectations, we will find it. But, if there's a major roadblock on the bumpy road to long-lasting love, it ought not to be the differences between the genders. Put the blame where it belongs: on stress. When individual stress is significantly reduced, relationship stress plummets, too. When we build into our relationships ways of relieving the stress each partner brings home, whatever differences there are between us as men and women fade to near insignificance. When stress is not a factor, our differences can actually become a major source of mutual fulfillment.

Men and women don't complain about their partners when they're feeling good. Problems and demands only emerge when one or both partners are under stress. Even our unrealistic expectations emerge mostly as an attempt to get our partner's help in lowering our stress. With a new, hormonally-based understanding of how men and women experience and cope with stress, we know that the instigator in most misunderstandings and arguments is not Tom or Nancy themselves, but a biochemical substance called cortisol. It's the stress hormone we were talking about earlier in this book. That's the real enemy.

You know how people with rocky relationships sometimes say, "It's not you, honey; it's me"? This is one instance where it's true. The problem is never just our partner's inability to cope with stress;

When we reduce our stress levels, gender differences don't matter so much.

it's often at least partly our own stress that's at fault. By learning to cope with our own stress, we'll be better equipped to help a partner deal with his or hers. By making the effort to see the world through his or her eyes, each of us can let go of our unrealistic demands and expectations. And that's how we find the feelings of acceptance, trust, and appreciation that are so much a part of what we call "real love."

With new tools and insights about what a woman needs, a man can help her cope with her new sources of stress without adding to his own stress. A man can provide the domestic/communicative/romantic support a woman craves, but in a manner that is quite different from what she was expecting—yet very suitable for both their needs.

The woman, as well, can learn ways to lower her partner's stress by helping him feel successful in helping her. Certainly a man needs domestic support, positive communication, and romance, but more important to him and his stress levels is the feeling of having been successful in providing some measure of fulfillment for her.

Finding ways to give a man the message that he is successful in providing for his woman's fulfillment is not the same as sacrificing for him. She's not required to give up her needs just to avoid being demanding of him. Women today truly need their men and whatever help they can provide. The problem is, women don't always know how to ask for support and assistance in a way that is realistic for his gender and appreciative of his efforts. When her expectations are realistic and he can meet them, he feels successful and his stress is relieved. Supporting him in this way doesn't require of a woman any sacrifice other than giving up her unrealistic notions of what her man "should be," and instead choosing to work with how men truly are. This is a formula that works in a relationship. It's also what real love is all about.

I remember a moment about six years into my own marriage with Bonnie when this became very clear. After a particularly great love-making experience I commented, "That was as good as it was in the beginning." I will always remember her response. She said it was better than in the beginning. Why? "Because now you've seen the best of me and the worst of me and you still adore me! That," she said, "is real love."

That day, Bonnie helped me realize that love was not just fulfilling some fantasy of perfection, where every need is met. Instead, it's sharing a life in which each of us strives to meet the other's needs as best we can. Forgiving our partners for their mistakes and accepting their limitations can be just as fulfilling as appreciating their many gifts and successes.

Hard-Wired to be Different

So, how do we get to this place of acceptance and appreciation? The first step is to acknowledge that men and women are actually hard-wired to be different. However we were parented and whatever way the world has treated us, our differences are predominantly of the brain-and-biochemical sorts. Understanding these hard-wired differences help us release our unrealistic expectations and accept that men are always going to be men, and women are always going to be women. When we first begin our explorations together, the differences can seem like walls that need to be vaulted or knocked down. But once we not only know, but appreciate the yin and the yang of our separate but shared existence, it becomes clear that men and women are perfect complements to one another. We were indeed made for one another.

Too many couples never come close to this sort of awakening. Things derail early in dating, at the time of commitment, or later, when marriage begins to trend toward divorce. Couples that don't begin early to fill a marital toolbox with ways of kindling romance, improving communication, and asking one another for help eventually grow apart. And when the split occurs, these are the reasons we hear:

"We were just too different to make the relationship work."

"He was just too stubborn and wouldn't change."

"She was too needy. Everything was always about her."

"Talk about self-centered: He didn't care at all about me or my feelings."

"Whatever I did was never enough. There was always something I did wrong."

"He was afraid of intimacy, and every time we started to get closer, he would pull away."

"Everything was fine until he changed."

"I was her project. She was always trying to change me."

"Gradually, the kids became more important to her than I was."

"Work was all he cared about."

"I felt completely controlled and manipulated."

"It never felt safe to open up."

"She's so emotional. It just wore me out."

"He never listens to me. All he wants to do is solve my problems."

At the heart of each statement above is a good-sized helping of misunderstanding or misinterpretation. These are people who haven't understood their partners, much less accepted them. No wonder it became too painful for them to stay together. Married or simply dating, how can we share our time with someone who doesn't know us and hasn't cared enough to try?

The successful couples, the ones who stay happily married year after year, often report that they long ago gave up trying to change one another. This kind of acceptance doesn't make either one of them a doormat for the other; rather, it's the foundation on which lasting love is built. With differences acknowledged but largely set aside, both parties are then free to work together to get what each wants and needs most out of life and love. It's not an easy road and it never will be, but our newfound understanding of the effect of hormones on our love, life, and happiness has made it easier to take the first steps. At least now we know why Venus and Mars are so dissimilar, right?

Understanding our Brain Differences

As we have discussed throughout this book, one of the biggest differences between men and women is how we respond to stress. Men tend to shift gears and forget their problems, while women seek to connect and share problems. This one simple distinction, more than any other gender difference, can wreak havoc in a relationship if it is not properly understood and dealt with. Tempting as it may be to see our differing stress-management practices as a problem, we must instead see them as among the "givens" in life. In fact, the bigger problems arise when we try to change our partner, to make him or her handle stress the way we do. It just doesn't work.

How we cope with stress is a direct expression of our brain's hard-wiring. As we saw in the last chapter, a man's brain typically has less connective tissue than a woman's. When a woman uses a part of the brain, other parts of the brain become simultaneously activated as well. When a man uses a part of the brain, to a great extent, there is blood flow solely to that part. The rest sits relatively idle until needed.

This is why men tend to do one thing at a time, while women multi-task. It's also why a man might forget to bring home the milk when he's busy thinking about work. Does this make a man uncaring? Without an understanding of how men's brains work, you might think so.

The neuron-rich brain of a woman has many more connections between the left side and the right side, so she literally has a lot going on at any given moment. Under stress she will have a greater tendency to get over-stimulated and overwhelmed. Does this make her emotionally weak? Without an understanding of how her brain is put together, you might jump to that conclusion. You might also consider her unforgiving when, under stress, she reminds you of every mistake you've ever made. But it's not because she's vindictive. It's just that her hippocampus, the memory center of the brain, literally remembers every mistake you've ever made. But there's a flip side: That amazing memory of hers will also remember every wonderful thing you've done, too—as soon as she's had a chance to relieve her stress.

Now, you may be wondering if I believe in gender differences so strongly that I can't see the exceptions to the rule. The answer is no. For example, I know that many men can multi-task. Take a male TV director. He does many things at once—calling the shots for three cameras, blocking out the movements of five or six actors, and listening to lines from the set while also hearing his technical director through his headset. But a woman TV director would do all the same things and still have brain cells working on what to serve for dinner, where to get a cake for her son's birthday party, and what to wear when she and her husband celebrate their anniversary. By way of contrast, the male TV director could well become so focused on work tasks that he could forget even big stuff, like his son's baseball game, or even his own wife's birthday.

Women's brains are wired for multi-tasking. Men's brains focus best on one task at a time.

Let's see if we can shed just a bit more light on how men and women cope with stress in different ways as the result of brain structure. The philosopher Plato observed that the brain had two hemispheres—one for serious matters and one for fun. He believed that the fun side was there to allow the serious side to rest.

Where men are concerned, Plato was right.

When a man shifts from engaging his left brain to using his right brain, automatically his stress begins to disappear. He can do it in a snap, no sweat. And the gear shift automatically starts his body rebuilding his stress-reducing testosterone stores.

Women don't have this luxury. Because the two sides of the brain are so connected, she never forgets her responsibilities—not even if she's deep in the midst of painting a picture or skiing down a slope. This puts a new perspective on it, doesn't it, when she objects to being told to "just forget about it"?

And here we have a great example of why men and women, though different, are so well-suited for one another: While he relaxes and forgets, in order to release his stress, the woman remembers. When he lets go, she holds on. And it goes the opposite direction, too. When a woman becomes overwhelmed by her over-taxed brain, the man's singular focus—if accompanied by love and understanding—can calm her and help her rebuild her stress-reducing oxytocin levels.

What we have here is proof of the old saying, "A woman's work is never done." The responsible side of her brain literally doesn't turn off. In fact, when Plato talked about the important function of fun or recreation, he wasn't even including women. Good that he didn't, because it simply doesn't work for a woman to become like a man. She can't relax and forget the

Our differently-wired brains can work to complement each other.

problems of her day simply because she or her man might want her to. Women cope with stress by taking time to share their problems and participate in oxytocin-stimulating activities. She doesn't forget. And, in a similar way, it doesn't work for a man to become more like a woman. He's not going to give up the cave and multi-task his way to stress-relieving satisfaction.

The important distinctions in our hard-wiring are real, and if we accept them, it not only helps us to interpret our partners in a more positive light, it also frees us from any expectation that they should think, feel, and act as we do. In fact, I'd go so far as to say that expecting to find similarities between men and women is one of the main reasons that Venus is on fire and Mars is on ice. Women think they want a man to be more like a woman, but really, what women need is to find new ways to cope with the new stress of living in a testosterone-dominated world. Instead of changing men, women need help to bring more oxytocin-producing activities into their lives. If they can't find the stress-reducers they need, they will only drive their men deeper into the cave for longer periods of time.

Back to the Future

If real love is what we're after, we must take a clear-eyed look at the destabilizing changes that have occurred in our relationships as we have advanced socially and economically. To the extent that these changes have caused some blurring in our roles—women in the workplace, men striving to get better in touch with their feminine side—we must find ways of bringing roles back into the sharper focus of an earlier era. I'm not talking about rolling back changes that were undeniably advances, especially for women. But I am encouraging all of us to remind ourselves that men being men is a good thing. And women being women is—well, to me, it's far beyond just being good. Our world just doesn't work without women being who they are.

Women are the custodians of love, family, and relationships. When women stop being women, I don't think it's an exaggeration to say we are all lost. Women remind men of what's important in life. Women hold the wisdom of the heart and inspire men to act from their hearts. Men can have a great vision of where they want to go in life, but women help men get there by providing them a solid grounding in what is most important. If women become too much like men, men lose purpose, meaning, and inspiration in life.

But it's also problematic for relationships when men aren't fully men. We have been led astray, I think, by the belief that men should respond to the new work-caused stresses bearing down on women by taking on some of her role at home. Due to differences in brain structure and hormonal makeup, men just don't change as easily as women do, so they're set up for failure and frustration right from the beginning. And even when there is some success for men who try to expand their role, the effort often backfires. A cultural sex change seems great in theory, but it seldom seems to produce a better relationship.

Often women lose their attraction to men who take on more of the traditionally-feminine responsibilities around the house. Women think they want men to see the mess, handle some of the shopping, and give the kids their baths, but when men do, some of the spark in the relationship seems to dim. It's even worse if he starts to talk about his feelings. Sometimes that causes the dreaded role reversal we discussed earlier in the book.

As a counselor, these are some of the things I often hear in such a situation:

> "I didn't realize he was so sensitive. I feel like I have to walk on eggshells so I don't hurt his feelings. I love him, but now I feel I need to protect him."

> "I'm just not turned on to him anymore. I want to be friends, but not lovers."

> "I feel bad saying this, but I really don't care about all his needs. It used to be that he was interested in me, but now everything is about how he feels."

"We've switched places. He wants to talk all the time and I just want to get away."

"He seems moody and depressed all the time. Now he's just another part of my life I need to worry about."

"It sure doesn't help me if he's going to end up more be stressed-out than me."

Certainly a man in touch with his feelings is attractive, but his sensitive side has to be balanced with a masculine strength and confidence. When women say they want a more "sensitive man," what they're really looking for is a man who will be sensitive to their feelings and respectful of their needs. Men can do this without becoming women.

Still, the biggest problem in modern relationships is not men who are not enough like women. It's women who have become too much like men.

Achieving equality in the workplace and winning the "war of the sexes" was a historic achievement, but it has left us with casualties. Some women who have sought financial independence have seen it come at a cost, ending up unmarried or divorced, and invariably, stressed. These tend to be the women who expect men to change at home, just as they themselves have had to change to function in a testosterone-dominated workaday world.

But, there are also women who have truly succeeded in the workplace, gaining much more than equal pay and status. They have also gained gender intelligence. And these are the women who can point the way for all others.

Equality between the sexes doesn't mean we can or should act the same way.

What is gender intelligence? It's what you're gaining by reading this book.

It's learning to understand the difference in hormones and brain structure that separates the sexes. And it's figuring out new ways of not just maintaining your love relationship, it's helping that relationship grow even in the face of so many new and sometimes confusing pressures.

Perhaps these women, the ones who succeeded in the workplace without ever denying themselves the right to be women, can guide us gradually to the future I envision: One where both men and women achieve loving relationships that grow not in spite of differences, but because of them.

Being equals, at work and at home, doesn't mean that we must be the same. Expecting people to blend into one perfect being, one perfect work culture, one perfect relationship, one perfect way of thinking, and feeling is to deny and disrespect our individuality. To truly give equal respect we must first recognize that we are different and support those differences. Respect is honoring who a person is and then being open to appreciate what they have to offer.

We Need One Another

Today's women don't like to think of themselves needing a man. But those who acknowledge that a need exists, even in an era of independent women, will find that they attract men like bees to honey. Why? It's simple. When a man is needed, he can make a difference. The more he can make a difference, the higher his testosterone levels go. If a man makes a good living and a woman needs extra financial support, then her receptiveness to him, and her potential to appreciate what he has to offer, makes her very attractive to him indeed.

I don't mean that the woman ought to be poorer or weaker to attract a man. It should simply mean that, in at least some area of her life, she should recognize a genuine need for male companionship.

This insight applies to all women, whether single or married, as they become more financially successful. Too often independence leaves women feeling they don't need a partner. When that's how they feel, they also feel less appreciation for what a partner has to offer. This is how expectations rise in women. This is also how he becomes dissatisfied, too. And then the downward spiral is hard to stop. As he gives less, she begins to expect more and more, making him more dissatisfied and her more demanding still.

> **When a woman realizes she needs a man, he then feels appreciated and loved.**

If the days of needing a man for survival and security are gone, what do women need from a man today? When I ask this question many women are stumped or resistant. They "want" to share their lives with someone, they say, but they don't "need" a man. They have become so testosterone-oriented that to need a man would make them feel not feminine but weak.

Needing a man is not weakness. It is what gives men a reason for living. It gives him an opportunity to make a difference and keeps his stress levels down by generating testosterone. Needing a man also stimulates more oxytocin and lowers a woman's stress levels. When a woman feels she can depend on someone for help, it provides a strong undercurrent of oxytocin production.

Eventually even strong and independent women admit to a variety of needs. Here is a list of the most common ones:

- She needs a man for romantic companionship.

- She needs a man for regular sex.

- She needs a man to feel special and loved.

- She needs a man simply for companionship. She doesn't want to come home to a big beautiful empty house or apartment.

- She needs a man for financial backup, someone who could support her if she couldn't work.

- She needs a man around because she feels safer.

- She needs to have a partner to share fun times with.

- She needs a partner to share with, someone who cares about her well-being.

- She needs a partner who misses her when they're apart.

- She needs a partner to create a family to come home to.

- She needs a Captain Emergency to fix things when they break. She doesn't want to do her own plumbing anymore.

- She needs a partner's support to go from good to great in her own career.

For some women, this is a new awareness, and it helps them to appreciate men. Women who appreciate men are attractive to men, which is good for a woman who may be looking for a partner. And if she's already married, her appreciation will be a testosterone-releasing event that makes him feel great. Understanding how much we need one another also helps a love relationship grow. Isn't this the reason that we cherish our partner after some sort of life-threatening scare? We see how much we need each other.

Getting What You Need in Romantic Relationships

Although we have covered in previous chapters men's and women's need in great detail, let's take some time to review the three kinds of support women are generally looking for, though in ways that are completely unrealistic. They are:

1. A domestic partner to share all of the homemaking and parenting responsibilities.

2. A person who is interested in sharing the feelings and events of his day with her.

3. A romantic lover who consistently thinks of ways to make her happy.

If a man were a woman, these three new requirements would be easy and automatic. But men are not women, and to expect his support in exactly this way would actually lower his testosterone levels and deplete him of whatever energy he has left.

There is hope, however. Women can get what they need, but not in the way expected. Understanding our different needs with greater gender intelligence help women to be more realistic in their expectations and provide missing information revealing to men how they can support their wives better. When our partners make sense to us, life becomes so much easier.

> Having realistic expectations for each other makes life a lot easier for couples.

In the beginning of a relationship, a man can give oxytocin-generating support to a woman, but eventually he'll run out of steam unless his own needs are met. Men need cave time to recover when they get home. If they go from one job to another they don't have enough time to recover.

It's a simple tradeoff. If he uses his cave time to do domestic work, he doesn't recover and fails to experience his romantic feelings that should emerge when his testosterone levels are higher and stress is low. When a woman is wanting more, she needs to prioritize what is most important for her and then ask for his support in a way that will work for him as well.

Let's first address how she can get what she needs in a way that can empower him as well, and then we'll discover how to best prioritize her needs to get the most support.

1. Getting More Domestic Help

When a woman requires specific domestic help, she should ask for it and not expect her man to automatically join her in caring about the chores the way a woman would. This is a common unrealistic expectation that raises a woman's stress levels. She assumes her partner doesn't care about her needs. Feeling unsupported around the house is the major cause of her stress. Even if he were to do nothing more, if she felt that he cared, her stress levels would drop.

When a man is not actively helping with mundane chores, he's waiting for an emergency. In many cases he's happy to help. He just doesn't know he's needed. At other times he wants to rest and conserve his energy for any emergency that may come up.

Men are happy to solve problems when she really needs a solution or when his problem solving will make her much happier. If he doesn't see it as a big deal, then why bother? If she's not asking, he concludes that it must not be that important. Just as it's difficult for women to ask for help, it's difficult for men to offer. Just as it can be challenging for her to determine how much to ask for without bothering him, it's a challenge for him to determine how much he can give without becoming burned out. When she asks for help in small increments and appreciates his support, they can both gradually overcome this new challenge in relationships.

> Men aren't wired for daily domestic duties, but emergency projects turn them on.

Gender intelligence studies at Harvard University have revealed that when people were working in a group cooperatively, men's stress levels went up while women's went down. When the tables were turned and men were working in a competitive manner, their stress levels went down while women's went up. When a man is competing he feels in control of his actions and his stress levels drop. But when he is cooperating his stress goes up. That's because he's not feeling in control. Men can cooperate, but this study makes clear what women need to know: It needs to be in ways where he is in control of himself and his time.

With this new insight, a woman can be more content to have her husband be her backup. He will be happy to occasionally take on projects when she's too tired, or handle immediate requests when she has an urgent need. But, to expect him to join in and share her daily routines as a helper would eventually exhaust him. When it comes to domestic work, think of a man as a sprinter and not a long distance runner. He is her Captain Emergency, whenever possible, conserving energy and rebuilding his testosterone for the emergencies.

2. Improving Communication

As we have seen, when women are looking for more in their relationship, it's generally because they aren't making enough oxytocin to relieve their stress. I've witnessed again and again a woman's feelings of dissatisfaction with her partner change to love and appreciation without him having to make any changes. She just needed to be heard, and suddenly, without anything in her outer world changing, she felt better. Communication is one of the most powerful oxytocin producers there is.

> A woman dreams of having a man who wants to hear her talk about her feelings and her day.

As we've seen, Venus Talks can help a man to fulfill her needs without it exhausting him. Although it isn't the kind of communication women fantasize about, it will produce the oxytocin she needs. This kind of support is similar to what therapists provide for their clients, because it is a one-sided sharing session. She talks, he listens.

Women need help with ways to ask for better communication in a way that doesn't turn men off. Men, meanwhile, often need more insight into how the things they unwittingly say can ruin a woman's mood and defeat the purpose of communication. Ultimately, a better understanding of why they fight and how to make up is helpful information for anyone. In my book, *Why Mars and Venus Collide*, I explore in much greater detail a variety of communication skills to give and get more of what you want in a relationship.

3. Creating Romance

At one time it was fine if after the honeymoon a man shifted his focus from his bride to his work as provider. In fact, it was deeply satisfying to women back then, because they knew that they were unable to support themselves and raise a family without his job. While this is what our mothers or grandmothers wanted and needed, it's not enough for most women today.

Women today long for romance because romance is a powerful oxytocin producer. That's why, as women have achieved more financial independence and success in the world of work, their romantic needs have increased dramatically. The more successful a woman is today, the higher the premium she puts on romance. The increased oxytocin produced by romance helps to reduce the stress of her work, which is largely testosterone-producing.

Successful women have a strong need for romance.

Instead of expecting a man to always think of romance, a woman needs to remember that he is from Mars and tends to think in terms of projects with a clear beginning and end. Once he has succeeded in being romantic even once, he thinks he's done. To make sure he continues to meet her romantic needs she must not expect him to always remember on his own. It certainly feels more romantic when he does it all without prompting, but if he doesn't, it's up to her to ask for what she wants in a friendly manner. Her odds of success will improve, however, if she doesn't try to achieve romance at the same time she's seeking domestic help and better communication.

Setting Priorities

When we look at the three kinds of additional support women are looking for, there's a clear and definite priority to them. For instance, a man can hire someone to help with her domestic work, he can even hire a therapist to listen to her feelings. But he can't hire someone to meet her romantic needs, so that must be the first priority within the relationship. I have a suggested approach for women seeking to work this priority list. But it doesn't start with getting more domestic help. My strategy starts with romance. My strategy may seem strange at first, but hear me out, I've seen it work again and again.

When seeking to get more romance from her man, a woman should start by telling him straight out that she doesn't expect him to do anything around the

> You can hire a house-keeper and a therapist, but you can't hire a romantic partner.

house if he feels too tired to do it. When he seems surprised, she can share her new insights regarding hormones and the ways that men recover from stress. Then, for several months she should be very old-fashioned about letting him take as much time as he wants for himself in the cave. She'll soon notice how much happier he is. In fact, when she finally does suggest that he plan a date for the two of them, he'll be so grateful for her acceptance of him and her appreciation of what he does for the family, that he'll be a new man. He'll feel that he's making a difference, which is how he felt back in courtship. And he'll plan a wonderfully romantic evening.

If the woman goes on the date determined to make him feel successful throughout the evening, she'll see him becoming more receptive to different kinds of romantic support she may be craving. Soon she'll feel happier and less overwhelmed. And he'll have more energy to become yet more attentive to her needs.

This scenario can provide an excellent prelude to the beginning of Venus Talks aimed at improving communication (Step 2 on our priority list). Suffused with her appreciation and his own sense of success, he'll be much more able to not only listen to her, but really hear her and understand what she's saying.

Then the couple can move to the third priority, which is enlisting the man's efforts around the house. Many women find that as long as their men feel they have enough energy, they're happy to take on more home projects.

This three-step program for prioritizing the support a woman needs from a man really works. Instead of getting lost in the day-to-day complaints and resentments of your relationship, you'll come out of this process with a new perspective and, quite likely, a relationship that ensures lifelong love. Instead of seeing ourselves on opposite sides of the table, each of us trying to get more from our partners, we can focus on getting each other more of what we need. In so doing, we find we have more—much more—to give our partners.

Chapter Nine takes us into the challenging change-of-life period, which isn't just the province of women with menopause. Men undergo their own hormonal changes. And if the couple hasn't solidified their ways of relating, it can prove to be a confusing and stressful time.

MENOPAUSE IS FROM VENUS, "MAN-O-PAUSE" IS FROM MARS

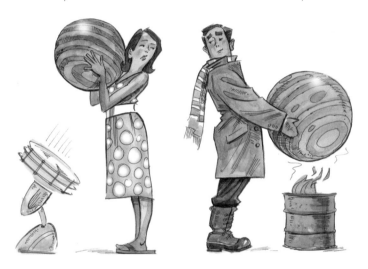

BOTH SEXES ARE AGING PREMATURELY AND THE CHANGE-OF-LIFE ERA IS MORE DIFFICULT— BOTH PHYSICALLY AND EMOTIONALLY.

There is a make-or-break time in the Mars-Venus relationship—a time when, fairly suddenly, love can become broken, even potentially irreparable. The woman becomes irritable and hard to please. The man becomes depressed and perhaps needy. Each of them, disillusioned by the new and unwelcome atmosphere of their relationship, begins to seek distance. Stress rises, health problems follow, and if they are not addressed with measures that improve nutrition, reduce blood sugar and ensure that both men and women are making the stress-reducing hormones they need, the quality of the relationship deteriorates rapidly.

This confusing time, so dangerous to love, occurs sometime between the ages of 40 and 55. It varies. It's related to the menopausal period that women used to call "the change of life." But that is not where the trouble begins, nor is it where it ends. What goes on for both men and women in midlife is far more complicated than that. It is indeed a change of life for both of them.

In this chapter we will look at what happens to both men and women as they near middle age. We will see how unrelieved stress, uncontrolled blood sugar and other issues are aging both sexes prematurely and making the change-of-life era more difficult—both physically and emotionally. By the end, you will understand how you can take action individually and as a couple to make this passage a period when love becomes stronger, not weaker. You will see that everything we have talked about thus far in this book provides the information you need to make the passage go as smoothly as possible.

> Middle age heralds a change of life for both men and women.

Our discussion must begin with a fairly thorough examination of the physical and emotional changes that occur between the ages of 40 and 55. You'll note right away that I'm not just talking about women and menopause. Men, too, experience a change of life. And we can't really make sense of the threat to the Mars-Venus relationship without talking about the couple as a system—a system that is, together, undergoing significant change.

Changing Together

You know about menopause. But do you know about "man-o-pause?" Between the ages of 40 and 55, men can experience a phenomenon similar to female menopause called andropause or, as I like to call it, man-o-pause. One of the big differences between these two stages of life is that menopause in women comes on relatively suddenly, at least when compared to man-o-pause in men. For men it is a gradual, year-by-year change that, in the Western world, begins when he is around 25 years old. Man-o-pause is characterized by a slowly diminishing level of testosterone. It usually isn't noticeable until a man reaches his forties or fifties.

But what's going on with men wouldn't seem to be natural, and it certainly isn't the pattern of testosterone loss that previous generations experienced. A recent World Health Organization report concluded that testosterone levels by age 70 are only 10 percent of what they were during a man's youth. In the history of humankind, this dramatic change is unprecedented. It suggests that there is something going on in life or in our environment, something we ought to be trying to change.

> Men today experience dramatic—and unprecedented—drops in testosterone as they age.

The situation is also unprecedented for women during menopause. Women have always undergone a physical and emotional shift from their childbearing to their non-childbearing years, but the common symptoms now associated with menopause were very rare years ago. In other countries, those same symptoms barely exist. Again, it seems to suggest that something's gone wrong.

A gradual decline in male and female hormones is a normal part of aging, but not to the extent it is experienced today. Sudden declines in sexuality, mood, and overall energy have not always been a symptom of getting older. We seem to be aging prematurely and not particularly well.

There is still much debate over whether man-o-pause is an actual change of life or if it is a disease state. After all, some men don't experience significant testosterone loss until their nineties. But such men are becoming a rarity, and what's surprising is, we hardly know it! When I tell an audience that a 40-year-old man today has the testosterone level of a 70-year-old man of just 30 years ago, jaws drop in disbelief. How could such a dramatic change happen so early in life? And, how could things be so different in just 30 years? The likely answer: Our current lifestyle, which has given rise to higher levels of stress, has created a widespread epidemic of low testosterone levels in men.

> Menopausal symptoms experienced by modern women were not at all common for our foremothers.

Women, too, are surprised to learn that hot flashes and other menopausal symptoms are unheard-of in different or less-developed cultures. Once such differences were attributed to diet, but research has gradually eliminated food as a factor. Now the focus is on lifestyle.

When Familiar Strategies Don't Work

We have already learned that higher testosterone levels are needed to help men cope with stress, and that one way a man can raise his testosterone level is to spend time in his cave, doing relaxing, non-stressful things. We have also seen that women restore their stress-reducing oxytocin levels by nurturing and receiving support for their nurturing. They deal with stress by talking with others and doing enjoyable things for themselves. But, today, for both men and women in their forties and fifties, it often seems that these techniques lose their potency.

For example, a woman could be sharing with her partner, but if she doesn't feel he is listening or that he cares, it will not produce much oxytocin. Indeed, his apparent apathy may make things even worse.

Similar things happen to men. As they age they find that whiling away time in the cave doesn't always ensure that they will adequately rebuild their testosterone levels. When they come out of the cave, they don't feel as refreshed as they once did. That's apparently because they don't feel successful; they don't feel that they are making a difference in their lives or anyone else's. Without that feeling of positive action and impact, much less testosterone is produced. What's more, if a man takes his cave time but feels that his wife resents him as being lazy, it could lower his testosterone levels even more.

When I'm confident that I have done my job of taking care of my wife and family successfully, and I then rest, my cave time rebuilds much more testosterone. Every man knows how great a well-deserved rest feels, and because it's healthy for him, this should be his experience every day. When a married man feels guilty that he is taking cave time, or feels that he doesn't deserve that time, then—even if he does take it—his testosterone level will not rebuild. Not only will his stress go unrelieved, it may actually increase.

Elevated levels of cortisol, the stress hormone, inhibit the production of testosterone. Without new and effective ways of coping with life's increasing stresses, and lacking sufficient support from a loving partner, men's bodies are limited in the amount of testosterone they can produce. And, gradually, over time, their testosterone levels will simply decline.

> When a man feels guilty about taking his cave time, his testosterone doesn't rebuild as it should.

I know plenty of men who are workaholics and don't take cave time. They age quickly, because they're using large quantities of testosterone each day without doing anything to replace it. I also know men who take cave time, but remain on ice. They have lost the loving connection with their wife, their family and most else.

Their testosterone levels decline because, lacking a feeling of being successful or of having made a sacrifice for a noble cause, their cave time isn't producing much testosterone. Making passionate love can undo some of the damage, because nothing is so powerful in stimulating testosterone production as a woman with a smile. In this way a man makes a difference for the woman he loves, and that, undoubtedly, is success!

Whether it is for the love he has made or the work he has done, feeling successful in the eyes of his woman is a mountaintop experience for a man. But, for too many men, this feeling of achievement seems always just out of reach. They complain to me that their wife has no idea what they do during the day and little or no appreciation of it. Men live to make their women happy, remember? The biggest damper on testosterone production is getting the message that, after all you have done, your partner is still not happy.

Why Women Aren't Happy

Women, too, have difficulties making enough stress-reducing hormones in their midlife years. When men don't understand all the little extra attentions women require today to cope with stress, oxytocin levels decline and stress levels continue to increase. The consequences are significant. With increasing stress levels, her adrenal gland becomes exhausted. Then, when menopause comes along, and it becomes time for the adrenal gland to take over for the ovaries, the adrenals are just not strong enough to make enough estrogen. Without sufficient estrogen, not even romance from her partner or improved communication will have much of an effect on her stress.

New research on oxytocin reveals that, in order for it to be effective in lowering stress levels, a woman must also have normal-for-her-age levels of estrogen. Estrogen is essential for oxytocin creation. Without these two hormones working together on her behalf, a woman begins to feel increasing dissatisfaction and unhappiness in her life. If her adrenal gland is exhausted and cannot produce enough estrogen to enable the production of oxytocin, then little that she or her partner does will have much effect on her mood. Whatever support she has enjoyed in the past to keep her oxytocin levels up is no longer enough. It just doesn't work anymore.

This is where the hormonal peculiarities of midlife begin to negatively impact a love relationship. When a woman enters menopause, a man is typically perplexed by her attitude. Suddenly his wife isn't satisfied by what he does for her, even though it's the same thing he's always done. From his perspective, nothing has changed except her response to him. Venus is on fire. During his wife's menopause, it's common for a man to tell me, "Suddenly, no matter what I do, it's never enough to make her happy." And when he says it, his feeling of defeat is painfully obvious. I can almost see him giving up.

Giving up only makes things worse in the relationship. He's encountered a problem he can't solve, and that dramatically lowers his testosterone levels. At the same time, his pulling away creates a problem for his wife—one that she may begin trying to solve. That raises her testosterone levels and does nothing to produce the oxytocin that would relieve her escalating levels of stress. But another strong possibility is that she, too, will begin to give up on the relationship. As she puts distance between herself and her man, she begins functioning ever more independently—and this, too, raises her testosterone levels as it lowers his. Her elevated

> Distancing may promote household peace, but it also reduces hormone levels and hastens aging.

testosterone levels also inhibit the adrenal gland's ability to produce estrogen, which means that she lacks sufficient estrogen to make stress-reducing oxytocin. In this way, the coping mechanism of distancing makes both partners grow old prematurely. Distancing quiets the rancor in the household, but it becomes a classic slippery slope toward decreased estrogen and oxytocin for her, and falling levels of testosterone for him.

As the slide continues, a middle-aged couple sees much of what constituted love and vitality in their relationship diminish. With decreasing testosterone levels the man become less interested in what his wife has to say, less interested in romance and less interested in helping around the house. Meanwhile, these changes in the man are causing the woman to lose her ability to counteract stress. Her major stimulator of oxytocin production has been his love and devoted interest. Without this support, she will chronically experience higher levels of stress. Throughout her thirties and early forties, even though she was stressed, her ovaries were making plenty of estrogen. During those childbearing years, in spite of an exhausted and stressed adrenal gland, she was able to make enough estrogen to continue benefiting from the oxytocin she produces. That's not the case in midlife.

When the ovaries suddenly stop making estrogen, a woman's stress levels dramatically rise, wreaking havoc with her moods and particularly her intimate relationships. The relationships that used to provide some measure of oxytocin support become unavailable or useless to her. Feeling abandoned and betrayed in her distress, she begins to feel increasingly overwhelmed, resentful, and exhausted. Then cortisol takes over and makes things even worse. Elevated levels of cortisol, the stress hormone, activate her emotional memory. Now she remembers all the good things she has done for her man over the years, minus any recollection or appreciation of what he has provided for her. She may wake up one morning and say to herself, "I have given and given and given—and gotten nothing back in return." Venus is now on fire, and it's not going to make anything any easier, certainly not her menopause.

What is Menopause?

At a purely physical level, menopause is usually defined as the cessation of a woman's menstrual cycle for a period for six months. Today, however, the term menopause is commonly applied to all of the undesirable symptoms that go along with this change of life. Common and unpleasant symptoms such as hot flashes, night sweats, mood swings and weight gain have come to be considered the symptoms of menopause. Too many women think that taking estrogen or progesterone supplements will fix things, but they won't—at least not entirely.

To be accurate, the symptoms of menopause are actually symptoms of hormonal imbalances and deficiencies that may—but don't have to—accompany menopause. Without enough oxytocin to lower stress levels, a woman reaches the age of menopause with an adrenal gland too taxed to take over the ovaries' job of making estrogen. And the lack of estrogen ensures that she won't make enough oxytocin to feel good. In fact, it can be like puberty all over again—wild swings in the production of estrogen, and progesterone, starting three to six years before a woman's last period. For a few women, it can start as early as age 35.

> In preparing for menopause, a woman's body may produce wild swings of estrogen and progesterone similar to puberty.

That's when the symptoms we have come to associate with menopause begin. But, remember, they are actually symptoms of hormone dysfunction. If the adrenal gland isn't too exhausted to pick up where the ovaries leave off in producing estrogen, a woman may not experience all of the supposed symptoms of menopause, and the ones she does experience may come in a milder form. Picking up where my previous list left off, these include: menstrual irregularities, breast tenderness, a declining interest in sex, brain fog, insomnia and fatigue. The vast majority of women today will experience their menopause in a two-to-10-year time frame, probably between their mid-forties to their mid-fifties. But some post-menopausal women report symptoms that continue for many years, some reporting hot flashes even into their sixties or seventies.

Although women have always had menopause, the symptoms above are relatively new. In fact, the cessation of the monthly menstrual period didn't always occur in a woman's forties and fifties. Even today, in some indigenous societies, women menstruate well into their eighties—just as men in their nineties sustain the testosterone levels of a young man. In these tribes, symptoms of andropause and menopause occur only rarely.

In our culture, whether the supposed symptoms of menopause are subtle and occasional or full-blown seems to depend on the hormonal health of the body. And, the impact on overall health and well-being can be significant. In addition to the symptoms we have already discussed, the below list includes still other symptoms, ones that can masquerade as hard-to-diagnose diseases and conditions:

- Acceleration of the aging process—wrinkles appear almost overnight
- Anxiety or panic attacks
- Bloating and indigestion, gas
- Increase in blood pressure

- Bone pain associated with osteoporosis
- Inability to breathe deeply
- Low energy
- Increased facial hair, particularly around the chin and upper lip
- Heart palpitations
- Cold feet or hot feet, particularly in bed at night
- Joint pain and muscle aches
- Lightheadedness, dizzy spells, vertigo
- Migraine headaches
- New food allergies or environmental sensitivities
- Urinary incontinence (worse when laughing or coughing)

While all of these symptoms are commonly attributed to menopause, they are actually the symptoms of adrenal fatigue, thyroid dysfunction, toxic liver congestion and Candida/yeast problems in the intestines. Let's look step by step at how these conditions arise:

1. Due to long-term stress and adrenal fatigue, the adrenal gland stops making an abundance of estrogen and progesterone. Instead, it makes the stress hormone, cortisol.

2. When cortisol levels are chronically high, the thyroid, which is designed to regulate the metabolism during non-stressful times, begins to under-function.

3. Elevated stress levels lead to cravings for junk foods that make our liver more toxic.

4. The byproduct of a more toxic body is the creation of fertile ground for the intestinal fungus Candida (yeast) to grow and permeate the terrain of our body. The yeast causes a variety of systemic problems, many of which are seen on the list above.

Here we can see in great detail how chronic stress has a cascading effect on our well-being or lack of it. It's stress, not ovary dysfunction, which produces many of the symptoms that occur alongside menopause. Here, too, is proof that women would have an easier time in menopause if they were doing more to keep stress levels down and organ function up, along with adequate support for the production of healthy, feel-good hormones. The closer we look at this, the more it's clear that menopause can be longer and less manageable if you're not healthy and relatively stress-free.

What is Man-O-Pause?

For men, man-o-pause is harder to peg. Its symptoms appear more gradually, as testosterone levels decline during most of a man's adult life. Remember, the rate of decline today is unprecedented, most likely resulting from high chronic stress levels and environmental toxins.

A man's symptoms of man-o-pause in many ways are surprisingly similar to those we associate with menopause. A decline in sexual interest, difficulty sleeping, weight gain, low energy, night sweats, mood changes, irritability, brain fog, depression and memory loss—these are all bad enough. It exasperates a man further to see himself losing strength, lean muscle mass, hair, and his passion for life even as he's gaining belly fat. He also often endures prostate enlargement, erectile dysfunction, aching joints and cardiovascular problems.

While these symptoms are attributed to man-o-pause, they are actually the side effects of low hormone levels due to high stress levels, liver congestion, decreasing thyroid function and intestinal problems caused by Candida/yeast. For men as for women, the solution to these problems begins with identifying the correct causes and working to eliminate them. Simply adding more of the missing hormones is not the right solution.

Finding Role Models for a Healthier Midlife

As I've traveled around the world, I've had the opportunity to visit a variety of cultures, including indigenous ones. In so doing, I've been struck by how many times I see men relaxing in the evening around the fire while women continue busying themselves with the necessities of life. Through talking and sharing with other females in a manner that stimulates the production of the stress-relieving hormone oxytocin, these women are able to sustain both their energy levels and their sense of well-being. While sitting around the fire, these men were letting both mind and body recover to be ready for the coming day. They were making testosterone.

I believe we can learn a lot about reducing the symptoms of man-o-pause and menopause by paying attention to these indigenous people and their ways of living. We can learn to respect the biochemical differences between the genders and honor both male and female roles, just as earlier cultures have. As I've said many times before, men and women are made for each other! Our differences complement one another and our differing strengths are what make it possible to build a relationship and a family together.

People living in indigenous cultures experience less stress because they respect the differences between men and women.

What indigenous people have seemed to know, and we're still learning, is that family groups and societies are more cohesive when gender-based strengths and weaknesses are accommodated. It's intuitive in these societies. Men sit at night to rest their bodies, because their muscles are tired from a day of physical labor. They don't know they're doing it to release their stress and rebuild their testosterone stores, but that's what they're doing. Women don't need to rest their muscles because, even if they're doing a significant amount of physical labor, they have the inborn stamina to keep going. In fact, research has proven that women's muscles have 75 percent more endurance power. So instead of sitting, the women go around crossing things off their to-do list and chatting with other women as they do it. They don't know that they're releasing stress and making oxytocin, but they are.

All they know is what works. In a Third World or underdeveloped culture, the effects of increasing numbers of women in the workforce haven't substantially changed domestic responsibilities or the ways in which women and men interact. And that's why they age without the kinds of side effects that we in Western culture experience.

Now, I'm not saying women—or men, for that matter—should go back to an earlier existence. I'm saying that an understanding of what worked in earlier days and still works in less-developed cultures can help us to better deal with the often confusing high-stress world we face today. And I can think of no time in life when mutual respect and gender-based understanding is more important than in midlife.

As we've seen in this chapter, in the 40 to 55 age group, our very health depends on men and women getting what they want and need from their relationships. Without sufficient stress-releasing oxytocin for women, and testosterone to counteract men's stress, each gender will go through its change of life with more emotional pain and physical maladies. The stakes are high, because the downside risks are the worst things imaginable: the loss of the love relationship, and perhaps even premature aging or an earlier death.

For both genders, the process of relieving stress is different, more complicated and, as we are beginning to see, in some ways more critical in the years between 40 and 55. Menopause and man-o-pause can make it harder to find and support one another. So, as we near the end of this chapter, let me highlight just two things that seem especially important in midlife relationships, from a biochemical point of view, of course:

More than ever, he needs time and space to recover. Just as a competition weightlifter can ignore his needs for recovery time and over-train, the middle-aged man hoping to help his partner at home with her domestic duties can unknowingly give his recovery needs short shrift. He may not know how much his testosterone levels have declined, and he may not understand that the usual amount of cave time won't always replenish his lost supplies. He needs to feel successful and appreciated to get the extra boost of testosterone he needs. And if he doesn't?

> A man needs sufficient rest and validation from his partner to keep producing testosterone.

Just as over-training in the gym is known to decrease muscle strength, lessen endurance, interfere with a good night's sleep and lower the libido, likewise a man's testosterone levels further decrease and his stress increases when he fails to get sufficient rest and validation. Not only does he become more exhausted than a woman would under similar circumstances, he becomes moody, grumpy, irritable or passive—in short, a man in misery who is miserable to be with.

What's more, he may become needy. Did you know that the average man at 58 makes more estrogen than his woman does? It's true, and the estrogen—combined with his continuing lack of testosterone—tends to make him more prone to sharing his woes with his woman. It's not the sort of change a woman welcomes.

Instead of being a source of support for his woman, this kind of man becomes yet another burden for her to carry.

More than ever, she needs to feel good in her relationship. A woman needs to trust that her partner cares for her as much as she cares for him. She needs continual messages that assure her of his love, understanding and respect. This kind of support directly boosts her female hormone levels, which in turn lowers her stress level. Without this reassurance, she may begin to feel rejected and, soon, depressed. This is because oxytocin decreases when we miss someone, experience a loss or breakup in a relationship, or feel alone, ignored, rejected, unsupported or unimportant.

To ensure that she doesn't begin to expect her man to be the sole support of her oxytocin production, it's more important than ever in midlife to encourage her to make other connections that enliven and reassure her. This will prevent her from becoming demanding of her man—which only serves to reduce his testosterone production and raise hers, resulting in even less stress relief for both of them. See Appendix A for a list one hundred oxytocin-producing activities a woman can engage in.

There is one other reason to encourage women to make outside connections: it counteracts any estrogen-fired neediness a woman may begin seeing in her man. When women claim their own space and seek the support they need, wherever it can be found, they avoid relying on their man too heavily and thus adding tension to a relationship that may already feel the strain of menopause and man-o-pause.

A strong network of friends helps a woman reduce the stresses of midlife.

Now we see how everything we have discussed thus far in the book comes into critical play in the midlife years. Next, we will begin looking at specific steps that both men and women can take to support healthy hormone production at any time in life. Learning how to lower stress levels to rebuild hormones requires more than just mutual understanding and appreciation of differing gender roles. We also need to learn how to maintain healthy blood-sugar levels, cleanse the body of toxic wastes and candida (yeast), and maintain a healthy regimen of diet, exercise, and regular sexual activity. These are the physical supports necessary to maintain hormonal balance, optimal brain function and bodily health right down to the cellular level. In Chapter 10, we will begin by introducing what I call super-foods, along with a set of practical solutions that provide immediate benefits.

I also encourage women to consider supplementing with high quality, natural products that support hormone production and relieve menopausal symptoms. There are a variety of supplements that can make a big difference right away. My favorite ingredients that I regularly recommend can be found in a line of products called WomenSense™. I recommend them because most women I've talked to find them effective. WomenSense™ is a complete line of products for women. Their MenoSense® product is great for reducing menopausal symptoms; EstroSense® promotes healthy estrogen/progesterone balance; ThyroSense® supports optimal thyroid health; and AdrenaSense® supports healthy adrenal gland function, reducing the impact of stress. These and similar helpful products can be found in natural health stores and online. If you would like more information on products that I recommend, go to BalancedPlanets.com.

CHAPTER 10

SUPER FUEL TO BALANCE THE PLANETS– NUTRITION FOR HEALTHY HORMONES

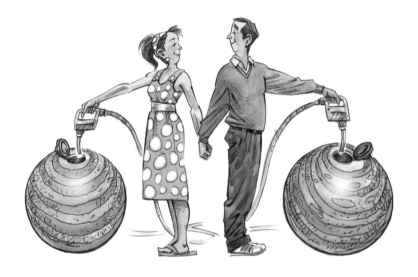

WE MUST FUEL OUR BODIES WITH THE NUTRIENTS NEEDED TO ACTIVATE OPTIMAL BRAIN FUNCTION AND BALANCE HORMONE PRODUCTION.

As we've learned in previous chapters, applying good relationship skills and making positive changes in our lifestyle stimulates the production of healthy brain chemicals and hormones. But there's still more we can do to help our brains regulate our stress response. We must fuel our bodies with the nutrients that are so essential to providing the physical foundation for our brains.

A prerequisite for good nutrition to work effectively is a steady supply of blood sugar. Steady blood sugar prevents spikes in cortisol, the stress hormone, thus preventing adrenal burnout and promoting the production of healthy hormones. Healthy blood sugar levels also provide fuel to make feel-good brain chemicals, such as dopamine, serotonin, endorphins, and gamma-aminobutyric acid (GABA). These brain chemicals help keep our stress levels lower. A steady supply of blood sugar is the key for healthy hormone production. Having the right nutrients opens the door.

Nutrients such as amino acids, omega-3 fats, B vitamins, and certain minerals provide the actual building blocks for producing brain chemicals. We can interact in our relationships to stimulate the anti-stress hormones. We can stabilize our blood sugar with PGX®, the amazing ingredient we discussed in Chapter Three. But without all the right nutrients, our body can't produce an abundance of feel-good brain chemicals and anti-stress hormones.

In the past, well-balanced meals provided all the nutrition we needed to stay healthy. Then, about 100 years ago, farmers started using industrial fertilizers that made it easier to grow crops without having to replenish the soil with minerals. These farming methods have greatly depleted minerals in the soil. As a result, our foods today are seriously deficient in the vital minerals that our grandparents took for granted. For example, it might take up to six heads of spinach today to equal the mineral content of one head of spinach of just 30 years ago which, by the way, was probably already deficient in nutrients.

During the past 40 years, the processed food industry has exploded, along with the growth of fast food restaurants. Processed foods are deficient in the natural fibers that would normally slow the release of sugar into the bloodstream. Sugar that's added to such products causes blood sugar levels to fluctuate even more. We not only get food deficient in minerals, vitamins, and good fats, but food that plays havoc with our blood sugar balance.

With farms becoming industries, more and more pesticides are used to reap the greatest profits. If pesticides kill the bugs that eat a crop, these same poisons wind up in our bodies when we eat the food. Such pesticides enter our digestive tract and can damage the intestinal cells needed to digest our meals.

Superfoods provide the nutrients we need for optimal health and vitality.

Because organic foods are grown without pesticides, they don't stress our intestines or immune system. Also, they will often have more nutrients. While this added nutrition is foundational for good health, I get my real nutrition from "superfoods" to achieve optimal health and vitality.

Superfoods are those that have been used by different cultures for thousands of years and are known for their extra nutritional benefits. They are super rich in amino acids, good fats, vitamins, minerals, and medicinal phytochemicals. Because they're generally not common, they're not yet grown with toxic pesticides and their quality hasn't been diminished by modern harvesting and processing techniques. They've also been shown over time to be free of adverse side effects.

I start each day with a cleansing drink made with superfoods known to help detoxify the body. Next, I take a delicious blended shake filled with a variety of

Superfoods dramatically accelerate any weight loss program.

nutritionally-dense superfoods, along with a testosterone builder. Then I finish up with a mineral supplement to compensate for the mineral-deficient food I'll eat during the day. I also try to take PGX® with every meal, to help keep my blood sugar balanced, and reduce the urge to snack between meals.

Over the years, I've refined and shared this routine with thousands of individuals and they, too, have noticed immediate benefits. Not only improved hormonal and blood sugar balance, and more energy for their relationships, but for those who were overweight, the added benefit of a quick but healthy weight loss.

This three-step program works because it doesn't require you to deprive yourself of anything. All you have to do is add the superfoods to your diet and your brain and body will work better. There are many superfoods, but now I'll just focus on the essentials.

—Step One—
Superfoods for Cleansing

Each day we're exposed to and assaulted by thousands of chemicals that can have a toxic effect on our bodies. Just as we need to regularly wash our hands, we need a practical solution to help our bodies remove toxins and impurities. To help my body cleanse itself of waste, harmful toxins and heavy metals, I prepare and drink a super cleansing drink each day. It's a combination of superfoods that work synergistically to effectively cleanse the body. Here are some ingredients I recommend, along with their benefits and suggested amounts:

Water, as a super cleanser, needs help to get all the toxins out. (8 oz.)

Sea salt provides all the trace minerals and helps the cells remove waste. (Just a pinch.)

Lemon is the master cleanser. In water, on an empty stomach, lemon stimulates the liver to produce bile. Bile cleans out toxins and activates the body's ability to burn fat for fuel. (The juice of half a lemon, or 1 oz.)

Aloe vera is an ancient cleansing remedy. It's an all-natural source of glutathione that reduces inflammation and helps the body remove toxic heavy metals that interfere with healthy brain function. (1 oz. of pure juice.)

Plant-sourced enzymes not only aid digestion, but help the body break down and remove toxins. (1 serving size.)

You can combine the individual ingredients together for a cleansing drink each morning, or they are already premixed in a product called Balanced Planets Refresh. All you have to do is add water.

A couple extra ingredients you may want to add are **Potassium citrate** (usually sold as a tablet), which helps the body's 70 trillion cells absorb more water and pump out toxic waste, and **acidophilus** (a beneficial "probiotic" found in yogurt and fermented foods) that can help protect the body against harmful bacteria, parasites, and fungi. In addition, it plays an important role in digestion. Acidophilus and other probiotics can also be purchased as supplements. A good multi-strain blend that can be consumed with food is best.

—Step Two—
The Superfoods Daily Shake

Each morning I make a shake filled with superfoods, some fresh fruit, and almonds or walnuts. These superfoods work synergistically to provide the extra nutrition our brains require to cope effectively with stress and to compensate for our nutritionally-deficient food supply. Here are the most powerful superfoods, with some of their benefits and suggested amounts (to easily make sense of the suggested amount, keep in mind that 4 g. is one teaspoon and 12 g. is one tablespoon):

Undenatured whey protein isn't processed with high temperatures that kill the enzymes like regular whey protein powders. Many people are allergic to milk products because they're pasteurized at high heat to lengthen shelf life. Undenatured whey protein contains all the amino acids in the proportions needed to make feel-good brain chemicals. It's also easily digested and assimilated. When protein is easily assimilated, large amounts aren't needed. Too much protein can interfere with serotonin production in women. And because extra protein converts to sugar, it can cause blood sugar spikes leading to increased hunger a few hours later. (One superfood shake should contain 12-18 g. of protein for men and 8-12 g. for women.)

Maca powder is derived from a root that grows in Peru at some of the highest altitudes on the planet. Maca is known to lower stress levels and, most importantly, increase the production of hormones. In my research with thousands of men and women, taking maca along with these other superfoods has stopped hot flashes in women and increased libido in men. It's good to gradually increase the dose to determine how much you need and to get accustomed to the flavor. (4-8 g.)

Goji berries most commonly grow in Tibet and Mongolia. When I was climbing mountains in Tibet, I noticed a lot of very old people who were also strong, vital, and happy. Several times a day they drank a tea made with hot water and goji berries. Research in China has shown that these berries help stabilize blood sugar. In addition they increase our ability to let in light. (They will literally brighten your day!) Natural sources of vitamin C have been proven to help restore exhausted adrenal glands as well as prevent age-related brain shrinkage. (A small handful is plenty.)

PGX® has proven to be the most effective natural substance for balancing blood sugar. I put it in my shakes to offset the possibility of the added fruit causing my blood sugar levels to rise too quickly. It slows the digestion of food, helping to ensure the normal and gradual release of sugar into the blood, and preventing me from experiencing feelings associated with low blood sugar later in the day. A healthy morning shake should ideally keep you from feeling hungry for four to five hours, and because PGX® expands in the stomach, it provides an even greater sense of fullness and satisfaction. (Experiment with what works best for you; 3-6 capsules, or 2-5 g. of the granules works for me.)

Cacao nibs are the pure source of chocolate. They are rich in magnesium and are an excellent source of iron. Beside containing a variety of nutrients to uplift your mood they also contain an amino acid called phenylethylamine (PEA) which gives rise to feelings of love and happiness. When we fall in love, for example, the brain produces an abundance of PEA. Taking PEA can help us relax, cope better with stress, and appreciate life's many opportunities to experience and share loving feelings. Both cacao and goji berries are super-concentrated sources of antioxidants, offering significantly higher amounts than other more well-known sources like blueberries. It's usually best to buy powdered cacao nibs or to grind the nibs in a coffee grinder before putting them in the shake. (4-12 g.)

Açai berries come from Brazil, where they are known to raise the metabolism to increase energy levels without the side effects of caffeine. While caffeine increases stress levels, açai berries lower them. Açai berries are also diuretics that cause you to excrete excessive fluids your body may accumulate. While you might feel thinner quickly, you may become dehydrated unless you take more water. Açai berries are usually taken in capsules, but some companies now offer a powder that can be added to a shake or to water, or juice drinks containing açai that can also be added to superfoods shakes. (A small handful is plenty.)

Coconut oil, a natural source of medium-chain triglycerides (MCTs), stimulates the body to burn more fat. You can eat plenty of this oil without worrying about getting fat. Not only does it increase your metabolism, it's not easily stored as body fat. Because MCTs are quickly absorbed and taken up by cells, they increase energy. Consequently they are often added to sports nutrition supplements. They help your body shift from the emergency state of sugar burning to the relaxed and longer lasting energy state of fat burning. Consuming more MCTs will make it much easier to go four to five hours between meals without unhealthy food cravings. You can add as much as you like to your shake. (Most people like from 8-24 g.)

Stevia is a sweetener, extracted from a South American herb, which has none of the negative side effects of sugar. It sweetens drinks and foods while also helping to stabilize blood sugar levels. It's very concentrated; too much can become bitter. (2-3 drops, or to taste. Sometimes it takes a little experimentation to find just the right amount to use.)

Molasses contains all the minerals that are stripped away from processed refined sugar. Like stevia, only a small amount is needed. High amounts of sugar can cause a spike in blood sugar levels. A problem with low amounts of sugar is that many people today have a degree of insulin resistance and can't fully absorb or benefit from small amounts of sugar. To compensate for this, I suggest a combined total of 2-3 teaspoons of dextrose and molasses. This will make sure the brain gets the fuel it needs, and as long as it's combined with good fats or PGX®, there's no risk of a blood sugar spike.

Each of these ingredients is available in most health food stores and online. There are also premixed shake powders that have many of these superfoods along with basic good proteins, fats, and carbs. One of my favorite superfood premixes is Balanced Planets Superfoods Daily. It tastes great and contains an abundance of high quality superfoods. Not all brands are of the same quality, so it's important to be selective about the source. I can personally vouch for the freshness and high quality of this one.

Even if you use premixed shakes, you can easily add extra amounts of maca, coconut oil, açai powder, goji berries, and cacao nibs or powder. Other great ingredients to add to your shake are ground flax, chia or hemp seeds because they contain high amounts of omega-3 oils, essential for the brain to make feel-good brain chemicals. In addition, they can reduce inflammation or pain in the body. An abundance of oils rich in omega-3s is needed to counter the excess omega-6 vegetable oil used in processed foods, and to help our cells effectively absorb nutrients. Because of their high omega-3 oil content, once ground these seeds have a short shelf life, and need to be kept fresh.

I have seven extra glass jars in my kitchen to hold these superfoods so I can add different amounts each time I make a shake. A little variety is good to get the nutrition we need. Some people like to buy all the ingredients separately and make their own favorite creations every day. We'd love to hear about your favorite creations, as well as your own experience using superfoods, at our online lifestyle magazine at MarsVenusLiving.com or at BalancedPlanets.com.

Superfood ingredients and premixed shake powders can be found at natural food stores.

—Step Three—

Oxytocin Booster to Calm Venus, and Testosterone Builder to Revive Mars

Either added to a shake or on its own, I recommend supplements designed specifically to boost oxytocin in women and testosterone in men. With all the stress of our modern lives, we quickly use up the nutrients necessary for balanced hormones. Women under stress in particular need an extra boost of the nutrients necessary to make oxytocin. Likewise, to cope with extra stress or simply aging, men can greatly benefit from a testosterone boost. My favorite formulas, available from BalancedPlanets.com either in softgel or powder form, contain many of my favorite ingredients, plus a few more: goji, açai, maca, cacao, PGX®, L-theanine, GABA, glycine, taurine, and apple pectin. The men's testosterone-building formula also contains Tongkat Ali while the women's oxytocin-boosting formula has 5-HTP added. More information on these formulas is available at BalancedPlanets.com.

Vital Elements for Venus and Mars

I also take a mineral supplement each day to provide my body and brain with the minerals that are missing in the good foods I eat. Mineral supplementation is also needed because when our bodies are in the sugar-burning stress mode we use up minerals much faster and lose them more rapidly from our kidneys. Since minerals are alkalinizing, mineral depletion leads to the accumulation of energy-robbing and health-destroying acids in our body. Superminerals are particularly good for energy, calm, focus and memory, but they are also needed for every function of the body. For example, magnesium has more than 300 known functions, including relaxing muscles, absorbing calcium into the bones, regulating thyroid function and metabolism, calming the brain, and ensuring bowel regularity. Without enough magnesium, all these functions of the body become less efficient.

It's not enough to just take minerals—they must be well-absorbed in order to work effectively. I take a combination of all the needed minerals in a form that will most effectively deliver them where they need to go. Orotate and citrate forms, where available, more effectively cross the blood/brain barrier and provide the brain with the support it needs. I personally prefer the orotate forms, although they can be quite expensive.

These super minerals also have an immediate calming effect on children who tend to be hyperactive or uncooperative. Here are the super minerals, along with some of their benefits and suggested amounts. I've provided a low to high dosing range; the higher dose is recommended for people under stress or seeking to support an exhausted adrenal gland:

Magnesium orotate or citrate helps ensure a healthy metabolism along with a relaxed brain and regular movement of the bowels. Women often need a bit more magnesium than men. (60-300 mg.)

Calcium orotate or citrate not only ensures stronger bones and provides extra energy, but also frees us from food cravings between meals or at night. (30-360 mg.)

Potassium citrate helps cells absorb oxygen and nutrients more efficiently. (20-120 mg.)

Zinc orotate or citrate helps men make testosterone, and promotes optimal brain function in both men and women. (20-60 mg.)

Chromium is used by the body to stabilize blood sugar and make hormones and brain chemicals work more effectively. (250-750 mg.)

Trace minerals, such as those found in Himalayan sea salt (mineral-rich deposits from ancient sea beds found deep in the Himalayan mountains) are required in tiny amounts for the body to function at its best. Most food is deficient in these trace minerals. (250-750 mcg.)

Another trace mineral of interest to me is **lithium orotate,** which I'll discuss in the next section when I talk about brain boosters for stressful times.

Following the three steps of the Balanced Planets Wellness Solution along with a little exercise is, in most cases, enough to activate optimal brain function and balance hormone production.

For adults and children who are anxious, stressed, depressed, hyperactive, or overly passive with little motivation to care for themselves or others, immediate benefits can be reaped by simply following these four steps twice a day. People soon begin to return to their authentic, motivated, energized, happy and confident selves. All the symptoms of increasing stress, fluctuating blood sugar levels and hormone deficiency begin to disappear in a matter of days. The results are even quicker for children.

Using the Balanced Planets Wellness Solution to Reduce Dependence on Antidepressants

I'm often asked if it's safe to follow the Balanced Planets Wellness Solution when taking medications, including antidepressants. The answer is simple. Think of superfoods as healthy meals, the superminerals as the minerals that would be in a healthy meal and the supercleanse as a super healthy lemonade. That's it. It is simply food.

If you're seeing health care professionals, most likely they will be unfamiliar with these superfoods. However, it's important to let them know what you've decided to do and ask if they have concerns about your decision. If they do, I highly recommend a second and even a third opinion from someone who is familiar with your medical treatment and also has studied superfoods.

In Chapter Three we talked about the widespread dependence on antidepressants today. Research has found that antidepressants suppress libido, increase weight gain and interfere with healthy hormone production. While there are other uncomfortable side effects that affect some people, almost all people who take antidepressants will immediately have an increase in cortisol levels. Antidepressants may sometimes give relief in the short run, but in the long run they produce unhealthy side effects.

For people who take antidepressants, but would like to go off them, I recommend additional supplements to make the transition easier. With antidepressants it's always important to make the shift slowly and under your doctor's supervision.

To begin the process of tapering off antidepressants, start following the Balanced Planets Wellness Solution twice a day. Once you're feeling better than you have in years, you may want to visit your doctor and explain that since you're eating better and feeling better, you'd like to begin cutting down on the antidepressants. It's important for your doctor to supervise this transition since he/she understands your particular condition.

More information for going off antidepressants, as well as bipolar medications, sleeping pills, Ritalin®, pain pills, non-prescribed street drugs, cigarettes, and alcohol is available in a free, downloadable e-book in the wellness section of MarsVenus.com.

Brain Boosters for Stressful Times

During stressful periods, our brains use nutrients faster to cope. Three very important supplements—iodine, L-theanine and lithium orotate—can be used to effectively avoid nutrient depletion.

Iodine, for Brain Power and Focus

More than 150 years ago, doctors recommended Lugol's solution—a solution of elemental iodine and potassium iodide in water, named after a French physician—for hundreds of conditions. It's well-known that iodine deficiency can cause a restless or foggy mind and that iodine deficiency in pregnant women is the most common cause of mental retardation in children worldwide.

Mothers with healthy iodine levels give birth to children with higher IQs. The seaweed-rich diet of an average Japanese woman contains 70 times more iodine than the average American diet. The children with the world's highest IQs are born in—you guessed it—Japan.

Iodine supplementation was stopped in the middle of the last century when drug companies started using radioactive iodine to stabilize their drugs. When the drugs were discovered to have dangerous side effects, it was blamed on the iodine. In fact, it was only radioactive iodine that caused side effects. Lugol's non-radioactive solution had no side effects, but lots of benefits. Because of the use of radioactive iodine, the use of iodine as a supplement got a bad reputation and went out of favor. Today, though, there is a resurgence of interest in iodine.

When choosing an iodine supplement, you should look for an all-natural seaweed extract rich in iodine, such as the Balanced Planets Seaweed Essentials, available in liquid or capsules. Even a small amount of iodine provides an immediate increase in the ability to focus without the adrenal stimulation of caffeine.

L-theanine, for Relaxation and Improved Focus

In Asia, a good green tea is coveted in much the same way a 100-year-old wine is treasured in France. The Chinese discovered hundreds of years ago that high-grade green tea is known to possess great healing power. Modern scientific research now backs this up. High-quality green tea has in high concentration a very special compound than can both calm and help focus the mind. L-theanine, a thoroughly-researched amino acid compound, helps the brain produce the feel-good brain chemicals dopamine, gamma-aminobutyric acid (GABA), and serotonin.

L-theanine has tremendous potential for calming, protecting , and restoring the brain. Researchers have found that L-theanine can induce deep states of relaxation without sedation; calm both premenstrual and menopausal symptoms; increase focused attention; improve learning; relieve nicotine addiction; and promote long, deep, and uninterrupted sleep. L-theanine is the only substance other than lithium proven to protect brain cells from neurotoxins.

L-theanine's calming effects in the brain can also help men relax so that the sexual experience is more extended. In addition, its ability to activate GABA in the brain helps men slow down and begin to appreciate the sensuality of the sexual loving experience. All the senses become heightened with increased GABA activity in the brain, helping people become less inhibited. While alcohol also has this effect, L-theanine doesn't cause liver damage or deplete the brain of oxygen.

> The calming effects of L-theanine can help relieve nicotine addiction as well as PMS symptoms.

By studying the firing of neurons in the brain, scientists discovered that L-theanine decaffeinates tea naturally. If a person takes about twice as much L-theanine as caffeine, the adverse effects of caffeine are completely blunted. If the taste of green tea doesn't appeal to you, you can also take an L-theanine pill before drinking a cup of coffee. You'll get all the benefits of caffeine—increased focus, clarity and alertness—without the nervousness.

This insight is particularly helpful for mothers of children who are taking drugs for attention deficit disorder (ADD) and attention deficit hyperactivity disorder (ADHD). When these drugs are effective, they're increasing dopamine levels in exactly the same manner as amphetamines. Prescribed ADD and ADHD drugs are amphetamines—the same as dangerous street drugs that are sold for getting high. There are other more natural ways to increase dopamine levels without harmful side effects.

When I need to really focus and think clearly (for example if I need to condense a two-hour lecture into only 30 minutes) I combine a couple shots of espresso with 200-400 mg. of L-theanine and 2-4 tsp. of raw sugar in 8 oz. of water. Espresso is better than plain brewed coffee because it's much less acidic. This combination is particularly helpful for anyone needing a pick-me-up for increased brain power.

Although teas high in L-theanine are very expensive, reasonably-priced supplements containing L-theanine are now available. A dose of 200-400 mg. a day may help you feel calmer and more focused. The same dose taken two to three times a day is recommended for those who suffer from anxiety.

Lithium Orotate, for Calming

Over the past eight years, I've helped people overcome depression, anxiety, and bipolar symptoms by taking superfoods combined with lithium orotate. Many people confuse the natural lithium orotate with the prescription drug, lithium carbonate. This confusion is unfortunate because it prevents millions of people from benefiting from this essential brain mineral.

Some users find that lithium orotate provides an automatic wave of calm and reduces stress by giving the brain the minerals it needs. The result is a natural sense of peace, not a manufactured altered drug state.

On a very physical level, lithium protects brain cells from dying prematurely from exposure to neurotoxins like corn syrup, MSG, and refined and artificial sweeteners. No other mineral has been known to have such a beneficial effect. Lithium has also been shown to restore and increase the gray matter in the brain—an astonishing feat.

Lithium orotate promotes a feeling of calmness while protecting our brain cells from neurotoxins.

Lithium orotate can also help our relationships by helping us let go of things that separate us from the ones we love. You may occasionally feel annoyed or irritated by something small your partner or a family member says, feels, does or doesn't do. On a good day, their behavior should be no big deal. On a stressful day, the memory of this annoying incident keeps coming back again and again, even though you want to let it go. You may find that a little lithium orotate will let you let it go and feel good again.

This amazing shift takes place easily if you're also getting all the nutrients you need. If you're not getting all the other superfoods required for optimal brain chemistry, simply taking more lithium orotate may not do the trick.

Even though it's a supermineral for the brain, lithium orotate has been erroneously linked to the uncomfortable and possible toxic side effects of prescription doses of lithium carbonate. To be clear, there is a world of difference between lithium carbonate and lithium orotate. Lithium orotate in small doses has been proven to be effective for some people. It's very important to use only very low doses, and to do so under the supervision of a health care professional.

With the new Mars Venus Relationship Skills we've discussed already, the Balanced Planets Wellness Solution, and these super-supplements to support optimal brain chemistry and hormone production, we have a lot more to look forward to as we continue to age. In the next chapter we'll explore the importance of a good night's sleep for maximum hormone production.

CHAPTER 11

VENUS AND MARS AT REST

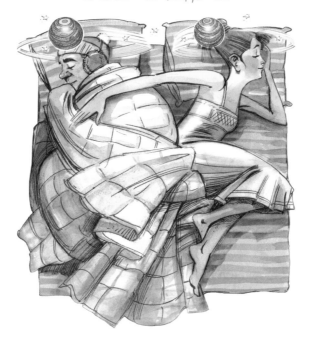

BETWEEN ONE-THIRD AND ONE-HALF
OF AMERICAN ADULTS HAVE INSOMNIA
OR COMPLAIN OF POOR SLEEP.

Sleep is the ultimate hormone producer. Indeed, a good night's sleep is absolutely necessary for restoring healthy hormones. Your body can usually adapt to missing a few hours of sleep, but chronic disturbances in sleep can dramatically interfere with hormone production. You may be getting all the right nutrition, applying all the best relationship skills, but without six to eight hours of sound sleep at night the body cannot make an abundance of healthy hormones. It's no coincidence that as people experience lower hormone levels, they sleep less. It then becomes a vicious cycle. Without enough sleep their body can't produce enough hormones and recover from the stresses of the day. Without the hormones, sleep suffers.

The brain needs to make an abundance of the hormone melatonin to immediately fall asleep and to stay asleep. In most cases, the proper daily routine with exercise and good nutrition will ensure a good night's sleep. Yet due to life's time-sensitive expectations, travel interruptions and schedule changes, it can be difficult to sustain a regular routine that supports a goodly amount of uninterrupted sleep. Natural supplements can help to quickly restore a healthy sleep routine. Then, once a good routine is established, it's often unnecessary to continue taking the supplements on a regular basis.

If your sleep cycle is off balance and your brain isn't making enough melatonin, a melatonin supplement may be your answer. Taking one to three milligrams of melatonin at bedtime will help most people fall asleep. This at least gives you a chance to start sleeping again on a regular schedule, which is usually enough to cause your body to begin making its own melatonin to sustain a healthy sleeping routine. Natural sleep is the ideal here; what we want is to help the body make its own melatonin. But to temporarily restore a good routine, supplementing with melatonin can be extremely helpful, and it doesn't carry the side effects of prescription sleeping pills.

> Natural supplements such as melatonin can help restore a restful sleep pattern.

Between one-third and one-half of American adults have insomnia or complain of poor sleep. A high percentage of these are women. As we've already explored, women experience higher stress levels today than men. In addition, women have eight times more blood flow in the emotional part of the brain during moderate stress. This increased blood flow in the brain requires the release of stored serotonin to calm the brain. When Venus is on fire, serotonin comes to her rescue, giving her brain calming relief. By the end of the day, if she has depleted her serotonin supplies, adequate supplies of the sleep hormone melatonin cannot be made.

How does the body make this necessary sleep hormone, melatonin? The process starts at sundown, when serotonin begins converting to melatonin. If there isn't enough serotonin left over from the day to convert into melatonin, the result is a person—usually a woman—who cannot fall asleep. Without melatonin her brain becomes overly active, preventing sleep. She will tend to go over her worries and her to-do list again and again. Eventually she may fall asleep from exhaustion, but unfortunately, she will be deprived of the hormone-stimulating benefits of a good night's sleep. This problem is often corrected with superfoods and nutrients, particularly lithium orotate.

Lithium orotate helps the brain make more serotonin and prevents dopamine levels from getting too high. When a woman is feeling overwhelmed or worried by something, her brain is usually making too much dopamine and not enough serotonin. With high chronic stress levels, men can also experience this imbalance, but it's not as common. That's because men's brains make serotonin 50 percent more efficiently than women, and men can store 50 percent more of it than women.

However, men can also have difficulty falling asleep, even in the presence of plenty of serotonin. With chronic stress or unstable blood sugar levels due to caffeine intake or a diet high in processed food, cortisol levels spike during the night. Increased cortisol levels have been shown to inhibit the conversion of serotonin to melatonin. In one study, nighttime psychological stress and the high cortisol levels associated with it produced a one- to two-hour delay in melatonin release. Drinking as little as two cups of coffee in the morning has also proven to delay the release of melatonin by several hours, thus promoting insomnia. Without enough melatonin, both men and women have difficulty falling asleep and/or staying asleep.

How Much Sleep do we Need?

Every night we usually pass through five phases of sleep: Stages 1 through 4 and REM (rapid eye movement, which usually corresponds to dreaming). We spend about 10 to 15 minutes in each stage. We cycle through the different stages like this: 1-2-3-4-3-2-REM, and then the cycle repeats. We spend almost 50 percent of our total sleep time in stage 2 sleep, about 20 percent in REM sleep and the remaining 30 percent in other stages. Infants are the exception. They spend about half of their slumber in REM sleep.

The first two sleep cycles each night contain relatively short REM periods and long periods of deep sleep (stages 3 and 4). If you go to sleep after midnight, these first two cycles are shorter with less deep sleep. Still, regardless of when you go to sleep, as the night progresses, REM (dreaming) sleep periods increase in length while deep sleep decreases. By morning, people spend nearly all their sleep time in stages 1, 2, and REM and no time in deep sleep.

> Deep sleep is crucial. It's particularly necessary to release growth hormones.

Deep sleep is crucial. It's particularly necessary to release growth hormones, and a lack of deep sleep is associated with depression in teens and adults. Besides the reams of sleep research that backs this up, I've seen this in my own life. After completing work on one of my books, I shifted from a few weeks of getting five hours of sleep a night to a relatively luxurious nine hours of sleep. After just one night on the new schedule it increased my strength in the gym by 10 percent. To me, the improved strength was dramatic, and I'm convinced it was the result of increased levels of growth hormone and testosterone—both stimulated by a good night's sleep.

Sufficient sleep is one of the most important factors in helping both men and women cope effectively with stress. The National Sleep Foundation in the United States maintains that seven to nine hours of sleep for adults is optimal, improving alertness, memory, problem solving and overall health, while also reducing the risk of accidents. A widely publicized 2003 study performed at the University of Pennsylvania School of Medicine, demonstrated that cognitive performance declines with six or fewer hours of sleep. Researchers at the University of Warwick and University College London have found that lack of sleep can more than double the risk of death from cardiovascular disease. Up to 90 percent of adults with depression are found to have sleep difficulties. Obesity is related to shortages of sleep, too. One hour less of total sleep nightly is associated with a two-fold increased risk of being overweight.

And there are still more data that prove sleep's irreplaceable role in maintaining a healthy mind/body connection. It's been shown that sleep—more specifically, deep sleep—dramatically affects growth hormone levels. Growth hormone is not just the hormone that determines your stature; it's also the hormone of longevity, the one that keeps you young and healthy by regenerating your cells. Increases in growth hormone are powerful enough to decrease all the symptoms of hormone deficiency in both men

> Long, deep sleep dramatically increases the body's level of hormones and restores health.

and women. Researchers found that during eight hours' sleep, men with a high percentage of deep sleep (average 24 percent) also had high growth hormone secretion, while subjects with a low percentage of deep sleep (average 9 percent) showed low growth hormone secretion.

Now let's look at how sleep influences your brain chemistry. During the stage of deep sleep, your body is able to break down proteins into the necessary amino acids to create feel-good brain chemicals. Tryptophan is extracted from proteins and moves into the brain to make serotonin, which relaxes the emotional part of the brain, which in turn relaxes the adrenal glands. Phenylalanine is extracted from proteins and moves into the brain to make dopamine, which gives us energy and motivation when we wake up. Glutamine is extracted from proteins and moves into the brain to make gamma-aminobutyric acid (GABA), which increases our creativity as well as our ability to enjoy our lives. These are the absolutely critical brain chemicals, the ones that relax the whole body, allowing the adrenal gland to rest and recover from the stresses of the day. The health of our mind/body connection rests on a good night's sleep and, in particular, getting enough deep sleep.

Establishing a Healthy Sleep Routine

When it comes to recovering from daily stress and helping the body make healthy hormones, it's not only how much you sleep or how deeply you sleep. It's when you go to sleep that makes the greatest difference, especially if it's deep sleep you're seeking. The earlier you go to bed, the more deep sleep your body experiences. The best sleep program is to go to bed around 10 p.m. and get up around 7 a.m. This gives you the possibility of eight to nine hours of rejuvenating sleep. Research reveals that the period of deep sleep is deeper and longer when achieved between 10 p.m. and midnight. Besides deep sleep, we need many hours of the other levels of sleep if we hope to cope with the psychological stresses in our lives.

Besides ensuring that you get enough sleep, a habit of going to bed around 10 p.m. allows you to benefit from your body's natural circadian rhythms. Circadian rhythms are regular changes in mental and physical characteristics that occur in the course of the day. (Circadian is Latin for "around the day.") Most of these rhythms are controlled by the body's biological clock and change with our exposure to the changing light of the day. These natural rhythms cause cortisol levels to rise and fall several times each day.

> A 10 p.m. bedtime matches the rhythms of our natural biological clock.

Cortisol levels are at their lowest around midnight and at their highest when it's time to face the day—between 6 a.m. and 8 a.m. They then take a 50 percent dip between 11 a.m. and 2 p.m. Then they slowly descend until they're at their lowest again around midnight. By adjusting our sleeping time according to these natural cycles we can gain the greatest benefit from sleep. This scientific insight supports the old saying, "Early to bed, early to rise, makes a man healthy, wealthy, and wise."

Night owls beware: If you go to bed late, deep sleep may be achieved, but it's shorter and not as deep. Your mind and body need the longest period of deep sleep possible if they're to most effectively recover from the stress of the day. Early birds, pat yourself on the back: By going to sleep early, when cortisol levels are naturally lower, your window of opportunity for deep sleep is much greater. As a result, more growth hormone is released.

Besides going to bed late, another obstacle to deep and sound sleep is unstable blood sugar levels. With unstable blood sugar levels due to increasing degrees of insulin resistance, blood sugar levels begin to drop around 3 a.m. As a result, cortisol levels spike in order to raise blood sugar levels. With bursts in cortisol, we wake up. High blood sugar levels, due to blood sugar fluctuations after dinner, may also cause insomnia. With this insight we can clearly understand the importance of balancing blood sugar levels for a good night's sleep.

Blood sugar fluctuations can interfere with falling asleep and staying asleep.

One of the biggest obstacles to benefiting from a good night's sleep is eating late at night. This causes insulin levels to rise for the next four hours, and that rise in insulin inhibits the release of growth hormone. Even if you were to go to bed early every night without fail, you'd miss out on some amount of growth hormone on nights that you ate within four hours of going to sleep.

For many people, waiting four hours after eating to go to bed is just impractical. Going to bed at 10 p.m. and having four hours to digest would mean you'd have to eat dinner before 6 p.m. If you need to eat later, there are ways to compensate. You could eat a lighter meal at night and avoid desserts and processed foods. So you don't feel deprived, have your fruits, desserts and processed foods around lunch time. If you do have carbohydrates for dinner like bread, rice or pasta, take PGX® (PolyGlycopleX®) to prevent insulin spikes overnight. Remember PGX® is a unique complex of water-soluble polysaccharides (plant fibers) that can help reduce blood sugar fluctuations.

All of this science is perhaps more than we need to understand, but I hope it has helped you begin to see why so many of us are so sick today, and why old traditions like not eating before bedtime and going to bed early have lasted so long. One of the biggest complaints people have today is feeling tired or sleepy during the day. One of the major causes of daytime fatigue, of course, is not getting all the benefits of a good night's sleep.

Besides blood sugar fluctuations, stress and eating at night, there are many other obstacles to a good night's sleep. Caffeinated drinks, such as coffee, soft drinks and energy drinks, along with certain drugs like diet pills and decongestants, stimulate parts of the brain and can cause insomnia, or at least difficulty getting to sleep. Many antidepressants have been known to suppress REM sleep. Heavy smokers often sleep very lightly and have reduced amounts of REM sleep. They also tend to wake up after three or four hours from nicotine withdrawal. Many people who suffer from insomnia try to solve the problem with alcohol, the so-called nightcap. While alcohol does help people fall into light sleep, it also robs them of REM and the deeper, more restorative stages of sleep. It keeps them in the lighter stages of sleep from which they are easily awakened.

Natural Supplements to Help You Sleep

Hundreds of people have told me that simply using the super-foods suggested in the Balanced Planets Wellness Solutions helped them to sleep better and longer. Even though I've followed this program for many years, I sometimes experience stress that keeps me awake. By staying up late, I then tend to sleep later, which then causes me to stay up later. To resume a healthier sleep cycle, I have found natural supplements to be very helpful. Some of these supplements can be taken every day to ensure good sleep, while others should only be used when needed to help restore a better sleeping routine.

A variety of health food store products will help you fall asleep at night. They generally contain a combination of the following ingredients:

Melatonin is the hormone that makes you drowsy and often puts you right to sleep. Your body makes it, but so do plants, from which it can be extracted and put in a pill. If you take too much melatonin you may feel drowsy in the morning, but drinking a couple glasses of water and getting some morning exercise can reduce this side effect. It's best to start with small amounts and increase until you find the amount that works for you. If you have 3 mg. pills, for example, you can always break them into smaller pieces and start with less. If you find yourself waking up in the night, don't take more melatonin or you'll feel groggy when you awaken in the morning.

5-HTP is an all-natural amino acid supplement that converts straight into serotonin in the brain. By taking this at night, you'll have a more abundant supply of serotonin to elevate your mood. Some studies have demonstrated that 5-HTP alone will benefit users as much as prescription antidepressants with no side effects. While this sounds impressive, keep in mind that antidepressants only help 50 percent of the people who use them. In my experience helping thousands of men and women cope with depression, I have found that superfoods plus 5-HTP taken with lithium orotate and L-theanine offer very good results. It's also useful to know that 5-HTP is utilized by the brain to make melatonin. Taking a small amount of 5-HTP (25-50 mg.) along with melatonin can extend the action of melatonin further into the night and keep you asleep longer.

L-theanine, a unique amino acid found in green tea and now made in a purified form as a supplement, is emerging as the premier natural product that supports mental calmness and relaxation. When someone feels anxiety or worries a lot, 200-400 mg. of L-theanine two or three times a day will provide tremendous relief from nervous tension. The marvelous thing about L-theanine is that it doesn't cause drowsiness and doesn't interfere with complex tasks, such as driving or school work. This is the same compound that was so greatly revered by Japanese monks who consumed very special, L-theanine-rich tea in order to enhance their experience of meditation. This same high-grade and very expensive green tea is still used today in the famous Japanese tea ceremony. Many now call L-theanine the "Nirvana Factor" because of its almost magical ability to promote a blissful state of peace and serenity.

When taken before bed, 200-400 mg. of L-theanine will melt away stress within 20 minutes and help to improve the depth and quality of sleep. If you awaken in the middle of the night, L-theanine can calm your mind, relax your body and get you back to sleep without risking grogginess in the morning.

While these natural ingredients are very helpful to induce sleep, they should be used periodically rather than continuously. When I need extra help to sleep, I use a product from BalancedPlanets.com, called Mars at Rest, that has a combination of melatonin, 5-HTP and L-theanine in a perfect ratio and in a chewable tablet for rapid action. The reasoning behind this product is that melatonin helps to get you to sleep but doesn't keep you asleep, 5-HTP helps extend the effects of melatonin and L-theanine improves the quality of sleep. If I awaken in the middle of the night, I take another 200-400 mg. of L-theanine to relax my mind and get me back to sleep without the risk of morning grogginess. Venus Dreams for women is a similar formula, but with a little less melatonin. Ideally, these ingredients for sleep should only be used for a few days to a few weeks until your healthy sleeping pattern of going to bed early and getting up early is restored.

How Being "Grounded" can Aid Sleep

Is it possible that getting to sleep is just a matter of getting grounded? I'm persuaded that it just might be! Ten years ago while doing research on indigenous healing practices in India, I was told the secret to health and a good night's sleep was sleeping "grounded." I was instructed to drive a copper pole into the ground and connect it with a copper wire to a copper sheet on my bed. The copper sheet was placed at the bottom of my bed so my feet rested on it. I noticed that I did sleep better!

Later, I learned about Clinton Ober's research on grounding from Dr. Jeff Spencer. Dr. Spencer used Ober's grounding technology for eight years helping one of America's winning bicycle teams during the grueling three-week Tour de France races. By sleeping grounded, the athletes slept through the night despite high cortisol levels pumped up during the race. Using grounded sheets, their cortisol levels immediately dropped at night, resulting in much better sleep. New research on grounded and ungrounded rats reveals that grounding also promotes healthy blood sugar levels.

Clint Ober developed the technology now used in grounding pads that allow one to stay grounded in bed without a copper sheet grounded to the Earth with a copper pole. He created a bed pad that is woven with cotton and thin strands of silver to conduct electrons. The bed pad is then connected to the ground wire of the house by merely plugging it in. If your house doesn't have a three-plug outlet, it's not grounded. For this situation, Ober developed a small grounding pole that can be put into the ground with a wire that snaps on the bed pad. If just one part of the body rests on this pad, the whole body is grounded. It's an intriguing addition to our tools when it comes to getting good sleep. Grounding is an area of great interest to me, and in Appendix B you will find some fascinating facts on electromagnetic frequencies (EMFs) and some advice and how to stay grounded while sleeping.

You're Getting Very Sleepy...
Tips for Improving Sleep Patterns

Here is a list of suggestions you can follow to develop a healthy sleep pattern and improve sleep:

Take a comfortable bath for 40 minutes before bed. This is probably the most important suggestion on this list. A warm bath for 40 minutes has proven to increase circulation, relieve pain, reduce cortisol levels and calm the mind. It's a simple tool to ensure deep sleep. It's not only effective, it feels good, too! For a soothing atmosphere, light a few candles, turn off or lower the lights and put on some nice music or listen to a book on CD. Low-level light signals the brain to convert serotonin into melatonin to help you fall asleep.

> The anxiety of trying to sleep can raise cortisol levels and prevent the onset of sleep.

Don't consume caffeinated beverages after 10 a.m. Some people may need to restrict caffeine even further to ensure a good night's sleep.

Replace breakfast with the superfoods in the Balanced Planets Wellness Solution.

Don't eat after the sun goes down. Ideally, don't attempt to sleep until four hours after eating.

Go for a walk after your evening meal. A little exercise not only helps digestion, but also reduces insulin resistance so that insulin levels are low by the time you're ready for sleep. For thousands of years, people have walked after meals and now, unfortunately, we commonly sit in front of a TV instead.

Get a dog to inspire you to go for walks after dinner.

If you can't sleep, don't lie there tossing and turning. The anxiety of trying to sleep can raise cortisol levels and prevent the onset of sleep. Instead, read a book or do some super-easy exercise until you become tired.

Use the superfood PGX® with dinner to help stabilize cortisol fluctuations. Blood sugar fluctuations in the night stimulate spikes in cortisol, which wake us up.

If you're too tired to make love but you can't sleep, a quickie can definitely help the man and it can be a loving gift from his partner. As women get older the tables turn. If he takes the time to stimulate her sexually, it can also help her get to sleep.

If your partner snores or is very active moving around in bed, try sleeping for a while in a separate room or using soft ear plugs so you're not disturbed.

Make sure that your mattress and pillow are comfortable for you. You spend a third of your life in bed—a good mattress is a worthwhile investment.

Make sure you get plenty of light exposure during the day to stimulate serotonin levels. Turn down the lights after dinner so your brain begins converting serotonin into melatonin. Sitting in front of a bright computer screen at night can prevent this conversion. If you watch TV at night, turn down the lights and sit a good distance away from the screen.

Put on some background noise to prevent awakening from random noises in the night or from your partner's snoring or breathing. Natural background sound generators are inexpensive.

If your partner says you snore, and you're troubled by serious daytime drowsiness, consider getting evaluated for sleep apnea. When people with sleep apnea snore loudly, they frequently stop breathing during the night. Sleep apnea is especially common in overweight people and it promotes a dramatic increase in nighttime cortisol.

These are certainly a lot of suggestions, and any one of them alone might do the trick to help you sleep better and deeper. With better sleep, you'll not only produce sweet dreams, but also the hormones that are so important to staying healthy and happy.

CHAPTER 12

LOVE, SEX AND HAPPINESS

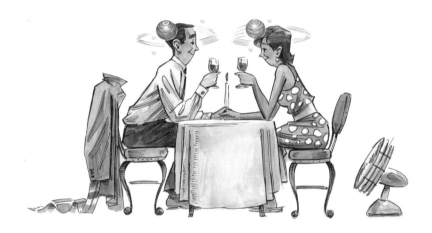

WHATEVER YOU'RE HOPING TO FIND IS WELL WITHIN YOUR REACH. YOU HAVE EVERYTHING YOU NEED, AND YOU ALWAYS DID.

So we've gotten to this point in the book, now, and you're thinking, "What's left, John? What else do I need to know to take this new hormonal knowledge and apply it to my Mars-Venus relationship?"

I'll answer that with just one sentence: You have everything you need, and you always did.

Think of that. You have always had at hand—or very near to it —each of the tools we have discussed in this book. All you have ever had to do is reach for them one by one, and you have done it simply by being open to new ideas and reading this book. I picture you placing your newfound knowledge of testosterone and oxytocin, of stress and cortisol, of cave time and nurturing, of Venus Talks, Mars Meetings, and Emergency Man, all in a box. You add the packing material of superfood nutrition, PGX®-controlled blood sugar, and restorative sleep, all for safekeeping. And what comes last is the wrapping and the bow.

In this final chapter we will look at love, sex, and happiness. This constellation of life goals contains other stars that we have already talked about, such as romance, communication, and healthy living. But, in this last chapter we will try to focus on the touch stars—the things that truly make a relationship a thing of beauty.

Love to Last

I will start with love, because love is where everything starts. It is what brings us together and keeps us together. In the beginning of a relationship, we ask for love from our partner and, ideally, the request comes from a place of loving ourselves. After we are together and committed to another person, the focus must shift to giving love, for love is the fuel that warms us, feeds us, and gives us energy for so much in life.

It is important, I think, to remember that in a mature relationship, love is not a feeling, but rather a way of being and, as some have said, it is a decision. If we are to love we must avoid the trap of behaving however we might happen to feel on any given day. That puts love on a seesaw with us; down one day and up the next!

Rather, to love someone while also maintaining our own love for ourselves, we must deliberately and wisely choose what we do in our relationship. At least as importantly, we must control how we respond to what our partner may do. After all, love doesn't grow from being adored. It grows when it persists and endures through times when we or our partner are difficult to love. Indeed, love thrives on challenges, especially those we address within our own hearts. When we struggle individually and together through issues such as gender differences, changing roles, and stress-filled days, there will be tension, but this tension builds strength. Like a muscle tensing and strengthening, our love becomes trained and toned. And it becomes something to rely on, an ever-present attitude that influences and organizes the way we live.

> We shouldn't give love to get what we need. Loving should be its own reward.

Ultimately, we should not love to get what we want or need. Love should be its own reward. I have a story that, for me, illustrates the point:

One Father's Day, at the end of a meal, my son-in-law began clearing the table and cleaning up the kitchen. My wife told him he didn't need to bother. He said, "But I'm happy to do it!"

I asked him why and he said, "When I drive home it will feel good knowing that Bonnie won't have to be bothered by the dishes."

This is a simple but clear example of love being its own reward. He knew Bonnie was tired after hosting the big party, and he simply felt good knowing that she would not have more work to do before going to bed. Not only would Bonnie feel good; he, too, would feel good knowing he had lightened her load.

To feel love as a result of our own deliberate actions and responses is a far greater experience than the love we feel in response to someone else's behaviors and actions toward us. As children, our feelings of love were dependent on how we were treated by others. As adults, though, we can only sustain love through genuinely making sacrifices to give our support.

But to give this support we must first master the art of supporting ourselves. It isn't so noble to make sacrifices for others if we neglect ourselves! We must learn to create our own fulfillment if we expect to be able to give others what they need, because only when we are fulfilled can we freely extend ourselves to others. Only when we are feeling good about ourselves can we expect our partners to take us from feeling good to feeling great.

Remember the 90 percent rule? As I've said, 90 percent of feeling good is entirely your responsibility. You gain your sense of well-being through the people and activities you bring into your life. Don't include your partner among these people, because she or he is a party to only the last 10 percent of your happiness. Ideally, that 10 percent is the best 10 percent, of course. But it's the add-on, the topping-off, if you will, of everything else you build into your life.

Keeping this in mind does a couple of things for the growth and enduring power of your love. First, it largely eliminates the blame game. You can't blame your partner for everything that's going wrong in your life, because he or she is a minor contributor, relatively speaking. Only 10 percent! Second, the 90 percent rule takes us right back to ownership of our well-being. Are we nourishing our bodies properly and sleeping well? Are we adding newness and challenge to our routine? Are we taking care to reduce the stress that complicates and weighs down all the good things in our life? If we aren't, we ought to find it very hard to blame our partners for our dissatisfaction.

> Your partner is only accountable for 10 percent of your well-being.

The culprit, the real troublemaker in our lives, is stress. That's where we should place the blame, and that should be the target that women and men share together in a relationship. Blaming our partners for our stress-based unhappiness has no value—in fact, it serves only to increase our stress. So, I hope that's one of your takeaways from this book: *Reducing stress is perhaps the single most important thing we can do for our own health and the health of our relationships.* Our detailed discussions of testosterone and oxytocin, and how men use the former and women the latter to reduce stress, should map the way to a healthier and happier life.

Unless we apply new and better strategies to stress relief, divorce and illness will continue to be our destiny. Cortisol, the stress hormone, becomes a poison within our system if not dealt with and dissipated. It's also at the heart of the regrettable tendency for men to become more passive and women more demanding, especially in midlife. You have learned some new techniques for reducing stress and rebuilding our feel-good hormones; now it's time to put the techniques to

> We must fulfill ourselves if we hope to give love without expectations or demands.

work—not once or twice, but day after day. It's not enough to simply react to changes in our lives and gender roles. We must take hold of our lives and repeatedly and dynamically make course corrections instead of going with the flow. You and your relationship don't have to be among the depressing statistics we encounter every day.

Another very important reason to cope with our individual stresses is to prepare the way for romantic and sexual behaviors. As we know, what comes automatically in the beginning of a relationship takes some conscious effort later on. To expect these things to just happen is to set ourselves up for failure or rejection. Bear in mind that sex and romance are not love. The two should go together, of course, but it is an utter fallacy to think, "Since he/she is not behaving romantically or sexually toward me, it must mean he/she doesn't love me." What it means, rather, is that these behaviors of love are not occurring, and it will require effort—*loving* effort—to bring them back.

Our eagerness for sex in the beginning of a relationship should not be just a fond memory. It ought to be a glimpse of what is possible in years to come—especially if we have taken care to overcome our inner resistance to both receiving love and support and increasing our pleasure in life. By opening ourselves to regular sex, we bring ourselves back to the people we were when we were younger and love was new. Regular sex will reduce stress, strengthen the love bond, and keep us healthy as we age.

Sex: The Cure for Much of What Ails Us

With its ability to reduce stress, improve health, and enhance communication, sex is—or ought to be—one of the most cherished gifts of a love relationship. Consider: Couples that have regular sex live longer with less disease. We can trace this back to hormones. Frequent sex raises the production of our feel-good hormones, testosterone for men and oxytocin for women. That's just the nature of sex. But when sex is combined with feelings of love and affection, the act triggers an even greater release of these heavenly hormones to lower our stress levels and regenerate our bodies.

We've all heard the "use-it-or-lose-it" admonition, and it's true. More sex makes us more interested in sex. With less sex, the hormones are not stimulated, and we become less interested. Sexual behavior then wanes. Still, just because we aren't interested in sex doesn't mean that we would receive no benefit from it. Quite the contrary! Do we stop exercising because it disinterests us? No, we make time for it and we encourage ourselves to get to the gym because we know it's good for us. Sex is like that, so... get to

Having sex regularly can be a disease fighter and a mood-booster.

the "gym" and start "working out!" Like exercise, sex becomes one of the great pleasures in life when we're "back in shape."

My book, Mars and Venus in the Bedroom, can be a handy reference if you're looking for more sex and greater satisfaction from it in your relationship. For the purposes of this book, I want to zero in on the hormonal aspects of a healthy sexual relationship. My goal is to help you understand that, along with good relationship skills, balanced nutrition and blood sugar, restorative sleep, and a basic hormonal understanding of the differences between men and women, sex is truly important to your health and well-being—both individually and as a couple. I want you to see that you should make it a priority in your lives together and that you should, if possible, increase the frequency of your sexual encounters. To do otherwise is, in my opinion, a missed opportunity if not a loss. Sex is one of the most powerful ways that a couple can achieve lowered stress and produce an abundance of healthy hormones.

Let me start by saying that it's not bad for you to have no sex, but an active sex life is really good for you. There is no right or wrong when it comes to how much sex is the right amount, but research would suggest that having sex at least once a week is the healthiest scenario for a man. Research reveals that when men have sex, their testosterone levels drop, only to gradually increase to a peak **Having more sex makes us interested in having more sex.** seven days later. This increase in testosterone represents his body's attempt to increase his motivation to have sex. If he doesn't have sex by the seventh day, then his testosterone levels drop back down and he loses interest. Loss of interest is not a problem, however, if a man is having sex more frequently than every seven days. To achieve maximal testosterone production, a man actually benefits from sex as frequently as every other day.

Women, too, benefit from regular sex. She produces her stress-relief hormone, oxytocin, in abundance as the result of having sex. In fact, I consider sex a super-oxytocin producer. It's the best oxytocin producer for her, short of childbirth or breast-feeding. The oxytocin released just before orgasm relaxes a woman's adrenal stress center and stimulates feel-good endorphins, just as sex does for men. A woman's post-sex oxytocin levels remain high while she is doing testosterone-stimulating work on the job, bringing her even more stress relief.

Regular Sex Reduces Cave Time

Sex is also a great way for a woman to get her man out of the cave without feeling guilty for reducing his opportunity to rebuild his stores of testosterone. Just anticipating sex helps with the production of his stress-reducing hormones. Following through, then, increases his production to greater levels, even as it spurs the production of her anti-stress hormones. Indeed, when Mars is on Ice, the most powerful way to melt that ice is by giving him positive messages regarding sex. Men who have regular sex and seldom worry about rejection have higher testosterone levels and spend less time in the cave.

Taking gender out of the equation, here are a few more of the many benefits that accrue from regular sex in your relationship:

- It increases life expectancy.
- It's a weight-reducing exercise that ranks with jogging.
- It leads to the release of DHEA, the hormone that enables the production of all other hormones.
- It can help with insomnia, depression, headaches, and pain management.

- It even promotes the production of collagen for younger looking skin.

And that's just part of the list. See my book, *Mars and Venus in the Bedroom*, for more.

There are only a few ways that sex can become a net negative in a relationship, and they tend to stem from how women treat the issue. Using a man's sexual approach as an opportunity to raise issues and expose conflict is not helpful. It makes a man feel rejected. Of course, a woman doesn't always see the problem she's created. She may say, "I need more romance to get in the mood. We used to go out on dates, but now we never go out ..." That's a fair statement and it's true for her, but her timing is poor. Also, as we have already discussed in this book, there are better ways to encourage your man to plan a date.

I have a couple of suggestions to offer for men and women seeking to get on the same page where sex is concerned. First, any partner who may not feel interested when the approach is made can make the "yes" conditional. Whether you call it a "quickie" as I do, or create some other euphemism for what you consider to be a limited form of sexual activity, there are ways of welcoming your partner's advance within your own terms. Also, you can each take the ambiguity out of the situation by signaling your interest in sex in a manner you both recognize. Maybe you say, "Let's have a glass of wine tonight." Or, maybe you literally light your partner's fire, as you'll see below!

Here are my top four strategies for establishing a healthier and more mutually beneficial sex practice in your relationship:

Light a candle: Candles can be a great way to communicate non-verbally your interest in sex. If, for example, a woman is interested, she lights her partner's candle. If he is receptive, he indicates this by lighting her candle. If he is not receptive at the time, he may choose not to respond, which simply means that his candle may be burning for a few days! But you can also make this technique more communicative, if you wish. How about a smaller candle for each of you to indicate an alternative proposal—perhaps a "quickie?" Both the signal and its meaning, of course, ought to be whatever works for the two of you.

Make a plan: To ensure that you're enjoying enough sex to achieve its benefits in your relationship, it's best to make a plan, possibly one that you can put on a calendar. If that sounds strange to you, I suspect it's because you're still thinking that sex is like romance at the beginning of a relationship, namely, that it happens automatically. But that's not true. Sex is like anything else you want to achieve—you have to set goals.

Nourish your sex life: Sex can stimulate the production of hormones and brain chemicals, but extra nutritional support can optimize your body's response—especially as your relationship begins to mature. As familiarity sets in, less dopamine is produced in the brain, so the addition of superfood supplements can make a welcome difference in your motivation as well as your follow-through. In my experience and from an abundance of testimonials, the regular use of the Balanced Planets Wellness Solution provides all the necessary nutrition to sustain a healthy sex life. But if you're looking for sex-specific supplements, there are many herbal sexual enhancers which have been used for centuries. Many of these seem to have some effectiveness, but this effectiveness is very dependent on the amounts used, as well as the quality and freshness of the ingredients. For best results, pick a supplement with a combination of herbs of documented effectiveness. In Appendix C you will find some suggestions for herbal supplements than can enhance desire, both men and women.

Treat yourself: According to legend, chocolate is a powerful love potion. Dating back to the Maya and Aztec cultures, people have used chocolate to enhance both sexual fulfillment and performance. Even today we need only a look at St. Valentine's Day to see how we associate chocolate with love. My favorite recipe for a sex-enhancing treat is to mix chocolate with equal amounts of each of the amino acids theanine, GABA, glycine, taurine and 5-HTP. A brief description of the benefits of each of these amino acids is in Appendix C. You can add guarana, a natural herbal stimulant, if you wish. These all-natural ingredients can be found at health food stores. If you prefer to skip the mixing, you can also purchase "functional chocolates," which slow men down as they give women additional help getting into the mood. These sorts of treats are available through many retailers, and at MarsVenus.com.

Creating Balance in our Lives

If you think about it, everything about this book and within it speaks to balance. We balance our relationships on the differences between the genders. We balance the release of hormones with time to rebuild our stores of hormones. We seek balance in what we eat, we work to keep our blood sugar in balance, and we even balance work with our non-work activities. Balance creates health and it also creates happiness. So I want to spend some more time with you talking about the 90 percent rule—the one that calls for your partner's contributions and influence to constitute no more than 10 percent of your life.

Over the years I have seen couples dive headlong into the Mars-Venus teachings, devoting considerable energy to learning and applying them to their lives. It's wonderful to see, and hugely gratifying to me to be making such an impact on so many lives and relationships. But there is a drawback to some of this zeal, and it's often seen in the form of an exaggerated focus on the relationship. Like a workaholic who's unable to keep the briefcase closed at night, these relationship-alcoholics have become overly invested in the quality of their marriage or love relationship. This comes at the neglect of other parts of who they are, and that's not good for them or for the relationship.

Relationships are enriched by all the life that occurs around them, not just within them! To sustain our health—be it physical, emotional or psychological—we need to attend to all our needs, not just the ones that pertain to a love relationship. Loving our partner and taking care of our most precious relationship are undeniably important goals, but that's just 10 percent of our lives. We have needs that ought to be met in other places, in other ways. *We need to take responsibility for our own happiness.*

Taking Responsibility for our Happiness

When we are in the honeymoon stage of a relationship, it is easy to be impervious to the many stresses in our lives. But once the newness of love has passed, we inevitably and gradually become vulnerable to the massive stresses in our lives. If we can just remember that our partners' loving actions and responses in the honeymoon stage were just a glimpse of how we can enjoy life together, we can create hope instead of despair. We can be motivated to take responsibility for our happiness without blaming our partners, freeing us to give our love unconditionally.

> Once the newness of love has passed, we become more vulnerable to the stresses in our lives.

Statistics show that after a divorce, men who remarry do so within three years, but women take an average of nine years. In addition, many more women than men simply *don't* remarry, feeling for various reasons that marriage is more trouble than it's worth. Particularly if they are financially independent, women may choose instead to live alone. In some cases they are happier than before, but that doesn't mean they're not missing out on another opportunity for happiness in the form of a new partner.

When I ask such women if their lives are better without a spouse, I'm often told, "I'm happier now because I finally learned how to make myself happy."

They aren't happier because they don't have to bother with a passive partner who resists giving to them. They are happier because they have given up expecting a man to make them happy and have finally taken responsibility for their own happiness. If they had known how to make themselves happy while in their marriage, they might still be married today.

Women who live alone and are happy have made this important adjustment. They have released their dependence on a man to be happy. The only downside for them is that they may be closing the door to the primary joy of being part of a couple: letting a romantic partner take them from happy to happier; from feeling good to feeling great.

18 Essential Sources of Love and Support

There are many places where men and women can look to find love and support outside their own love relationships, and it's important to be looking! By taking responsibility for nurturing and being nurtured in these other ways, we relieve our partners of an impossible burden—being our all and everything. Think of the following ideas and opportunities as "love vitamins." The romantic love our partner gives us is just one vitamin. If we are deficient in that vitamin, then taking it makes a huge difference in our health and well-being. But if we are deficient in all our other vitamins, then no matter how much our romantic partner gives, we will be too deficient to benefit.

1. Look to Yourself

Treating ourselves with kindness, respect, and compassion is the foundation of feeling good. Without this self-support, we depend too much upon our partners for our self-esteem. Think of the times our partner has criticized us for something we've said or done. If we're stressed or blue, even the smallest comment can easily be taken as a profound indictment.

> By finding love and support independent of our partners, we relieve them of solely supporting us.

But if we have taken good care of ourselves, we will either accept the criticism, recognizing its value, or brush it off as we choose.

One way to love yourself is to do for yourself things that you would do for someone you love. Another is to treat your body with extra care, getting sufficient exercise and nutrition. Not letting others mistreat you or cross your boundaries is still another way of loving yourself. The more you focus on finding ways to love yourself, the more you open the door for others to love you as well.

2. Look to Your Work and Coworkers

When we don't have meaningful work in our lives, we expect our partners to need us more and thus make our lives more fulfilled. Our romantic partner should never be a substitute for our need to make a difference in the world. It is very important that we feel in some way that we are contributing to the well-being of others. This makes us feel connected to the world with a sense of higher purpose.

> Our romantic partner can never be a substitute for our need to make the world better.

Serving, leading, and participating in a work setting all build our sense of self-worth. If we do not regularly experience being of value to the world beyond the four walls of our family home, we become too dependent on our partner to make us feel good. In turn, our partners feel defeated by our neediness and our ever-increasing demands.

3. Look to Rest, Recreation, Hobbies and Vacations

When we don't take time for relaxation and recreation, we may unfairly expect our partners to entertain us or make life entertaining. Then, when life becomes flat or boring we blame our partners instead of taking time out for fun on our own.

A woman needs regular vacations or little getaways to escape all the things that remind her of her responsibilities.

> Both men and women need occasional breaks from their responsibilities.

A cruise or a stay at a hotel or spa can be rejuvenating. But simply eating a delicious meal at a lovely restaurant can work wonders because she doesn't feel the pressure to prepare the menu, do the shopping, cook and then clean up. While these tasks can be a great source of fulfillment to her, she also needs a break from them.

A man typically needs some kind of regular recreation or hobby that helps him take his mind off work. If a man is so busy trying to earn a living that he comes home too exhausted to participate in the relationship, it is a sign that he needs to create some kind of hobby, something that has nothing to do with his line of business. This distraction will actually give him the support he needs to avoid exhaustion through work and, as a result, he will have more to give to his partner and children.

4. Look to Your Schedule

When you don't include time for yourself in your schedule, you will tend to feel that your partner is not taking enough time for you. Ideally, busy couples should sit together with a calendar and schedule time to spend together as well as time apart.

If you don't make time for yourself, don't expect your partner to.

When special times are scheduled and noted on the calendar, it gives a woman something to look forward to, which is a stress-reliever for her. For a man, scheduling is important because he easily overlooks taking time to enjoy his relationship. He gets too caught up in providing for his family and forgets to simply spend time with them. He doesn't realize how quickly time passes or how much his presence is needed and appreciated.

5. Look to Outside Help

With so much to do and so little time, it is unrealistic for couples to expect to be able to maintain their home the way their parents did—not without extra help, that is. Having more chores to do than

Hired help makes a big difference when couples are just too busy or overworked to do it all.

we have energy or time for, creates extra stress for both men and women. He should not expect her to do it all, nor should she expect him to exhaust himself trying to fulfill unrealistic expectations. Without obtaining extra help, they will both be too stressed out to feel good. Keep in mind that back when women handled all the cooking and cleaning, they were not working outside the home each day. Just as he needs a break at the end of his work day, she needs time to relax as well.

If women are to spend many hours outside the home earning money, then a portion of the family's earnings needs to be budgeted to hire household help, even if it's just a cleaning service. Given today's fast-paced life, stay-at-home moms can also benefit from paid assistance. Without this kind support, a woman can easily feel overwhelmed and then exert an unhealthy pressure on her partner for help. If he is already exhausted after his day at work, to expect more than he has the energy to give drives a wedge between them. Hired help can reduce the tension of partners who are spread too thinly.

6. Look to Your Priorities

Women have a tendency to take on too much. By prioritizing and focusing on what is most important to them, they will feel less compelled to do and be everything for everyone. The sense of urgency in their lives will diminish and oxytocin levels will soar.

A woman's toxic sense of urgency is certainly an act of caring, but it is rooted in a lack of trust. Deep down, she wonders whether she will be loved even if she is not what everyone wants her to be. But, when a woman allows everyone else set the priorities, she will soon come to believe that her partner is the one not making a priority—of her!

It's different for men. When men don't recognize or act in accordance with their priorities they become weak, moody, and passive. They may become temperamental when their wives don't live up to their expectations. Rather than

> When you are not making yourself a priority, you will begin to feel neglected in your relationship.

feeling compassionate, a man may become annoyed and irritated.

On Mars, taking action congruent with your priorities means keeping your word. If a man says he will do something, then he intends to follow through and do his very best to get the job done. If he can't do what he says, then he needs to adjust his thinking and make a new promise that he can deliver. This kind of integrity and determination releases a gush of testosterone and allows him to feel deeply satisfied when he takes his rest to rebuild testosterone.

For a man, delayed gratification or sacrifice strengthens his resolve and character. By prioritizing his actions to keep his promises, he is empowered to be his best self. When he doesn't make the necessary sacrifices to keep his promises, he lives as a victim to negativism, focusing on how others disappoint him by not keeping their promises. Unless he takes responsible action each day to set and meet his priorities, he will focus on the negative; namely, how his partner has disappointed him. He'll forget the many ways she has supported him.

7. Look to Your Friendships

There is nothing wrong with being best friends with your partner, as long as you have other friends as well. When we don't take time to create and nurture friendships, we unreasonably expect our partners to fill this void. The need for friendships must be met outside our intimate relationships, so as to prevent us from expecting too much from our partners. Friendships help stimulate the hormone oxytocin. Generally, a few friends are sufficient for a man, but because women tend to run out of oxytocin more readily, they generally need more friends.

> Without friendships, women expect men to be chatty and men expect women to be low maintenance.

Without enough supportive friends, women expect their partners to be chatty, like their girl friends, just as men will expect their partners to be more easy-going, like their buddies. These unrealistic expectations of their partners can create resentment and annoyance.

There is another factor to consider: the joy of coming home to one another. A healthy distance from your intimate partner can spark and sustain feelings of attraction. If spouses or lovers are together all the time, then there is no opportunity to experience the pleasure of coming together.

8. Look To Your Family Members

One of the biggest sources of stress today, particularly for women, is the fragmentation of the family. Family is certainly important for a man, but it's much more important for a woman, since it is a major producer of stress-reducing oxytocin.

Staying in touch and spending time with relatives is nurturing to the soul, because a part of knowing who we are is knowing where we came from. Family members ought to be our foundation in life, because aside from our partners, they are the only ones who offer us unconditional love. But even when they don't love us, they can be of value to us. By practicing acceptance of challenging family members, we also learn how to let go of the unrealistic expectations we may hold of our partners. If we neglect this need, we may become clingy or demanding with our partner, or perhaps even jealous of how they spend their time. Unconsciously, we may begin expecting our partner to parent us! This, of course, is life-threatening to a relationship.

> By accepting our parents and family members as they are, we are better able to accept ourselves and our partners.

9. Look to Spiritual Support and Inspiration

Not everyone incorporates spiritual practice into their lives. But those who feel a yearning to do so must fulfill their need. Without doing so, it is just another unmet need we inappropriately look to our partners to fill.

Even the non-spiritual among us need sources of inspiration. Simply spending time with people who have earned your respect and admiration can fit the bill. Association with people of like values reminds us of what is important to us. Without some form of inspiration in our lives, we deprive ourselves of a particularly rewarding type of personal growth.

> Unless we are inspired to grow, life becomes tiring and boring.

Reading good books by authors that we respect is another great source of inspiration. Listening to music—or even playing it ourselves—is inspiring as well.

10. Look to Special Occasions

Without special occasions, like family get-togethers, reunions, or community events, such as parades, fairs, weddings, dances, and public concerts, we put too much pressure on our intimate relationships to celebrate milestones and make us feel special.

When women have the opportunity to give of themselves freely at community events, and not because they are being paid, oxytocin is released. For men, testosterone is released when they feel their efforts to support others are being publicly appreciated or rewarded.

> We can't expect romance to do it all. Special occasions make us feel special.

Women, more so than men, need extra support to feel special. Inside the relationship, a special occasion is created whenever men make small, but considerate gestures like picking up her favorite takeout food or buying special sweets for her. These little things add up and they do make a big difference, but without the opportunities for unconditional giving that special gatherings outside the home provide, the little things will never be enough to satisfy her need to feel special.

Men feel special when they are welcomed by others and appreciated for their efforts. It's a special occasion for any man when the outside world recognizes a special moment or achievement in his life.

11. Look to Other Couples

Spending time with other couples gives a great boost to your relationship. It allows you to be in your partner's presence and hear and see them through the eyes and ears of others.

While spending time with other couples, we spontaneously tell old stories or describe what is going on in our life. Alone with our partners, we wouldn't normally bring these things up because our partner already knows about them. But, because your friends have not yet heard these stories or what is new in your life, a feeling of newness is stimulated.

> Seeing our partner through the perspective of others helps us let go of old notions of who our partner is and is not.

Talking about current events and the news while other couples are present also helps expand our perspective, and allows us to appreciate our partners' perspective even more. Hearing and seeing our partners through the perspective of others help us let go of old notions of who our partner is and is not.

There is one more great benefit to spending time with other couples. Conversation with the same person over the years tends to bring out only certain aspects of who we are. Conversation with others brings out different parts of our personality. This "newness" is then revealed to our partner as well.

12. Look to Continuing Education

A major source of newness in our lives is continued learning. It is the learning curve of a new relationship that stimulates so many heavenly hormones, particularly the sexual hormones that were so abundant in our adolescence. Learning new things not only creates healthy hormones, but it actually stimulates the growth of brain cells.

Taking a class at a local community college or attending a personal growth seminar can give our energy levels a huge lift. When we are learning new things, a new part of our self is emerging. This newness flows into our relationship and brings back the feelings we had when our relationship was new. Without partners infusing new learning into the relationship, we can easily become bored with marriage and even life itself. By taking classes and learning from others, a whole new world opens up to us, and, as a result, our relationship at home becomes more exciting.

> When we are learning new things, a new part of our self is emerging.

13. Look to Individual Therapy or Life Coaching

When we have unresolved issues from childhood, it is very important that we handle these matters separate from our partner. If you didn't get parental support from your parents, don't try to find it from your partner. Instead, consider seeing a therapist— therapy is a more appropriate way to nurture the need to make up for what was missing in your childhood.

By having private sessions, we have an opportunity to vent our thoughts and feelings, as well as to explore our goals and strategies without having to worry about hurting anyone or being held accountable for what we have said. So many relationships are ruined when people have no one but their partner to talk to. They either suppress their feelings by not talking things out, or they blurt out their thoughts and feelings at inappropriate times. Individual therapy or life coaching can be incredibly fulfilling. It also takes the burden off our partner to be our teacher, guide, and parent all wrapped up in one.

> Many relationships are harmed when people have no one else to talk to.

Therapy can also provide stability in life, for it allows us an opportunity to see ourselves more objectively. It is also particularly helpful to women, as talking produces oxytocin, their anti-stress hormone. Furthermore, when women anticipate being able to share how they feel with someone, the unrealistic desire to be fully understood by their partner evaporates. For men, talking with someone privately releases them from the need to keep everything inside to protect themselves from the real consequences in the work world of revealing their vulnerabilities.

14. Look to Some Kind of Support Group

One of the most powerful hormone stimulators in our lives can be a same-sex support group.

Women today are missing the hormonal stimulation that occurs when women share, communicate, commiserate and cooperate in a non-work oriented context. Just talking about what is going on in their lives without the intent to fix anyone or solve anything is one of the most practical things a woman can do to rebuild oxytocin levels. Even looking forward to these meetings and the support they will receive from other women sustains higher levels of stress-reducing hormones for days in advance.

> There are some things that only women— or only men—can understand.

The work world often gives men much of the support they need, but an all-male support group can give a man the opportunity to express what's going on in his life without having to edit himself. Going out to the movies with a friend, being on a sports team or simply going to a sporting event with the guys can also be very testosterone-stimulating.

Interestingly enough, being with women or with his female partner for a long time can actually lower a man's testosterone levels. A sign that this may be happening is when he begins to feel tired in his woman's presence or when he feels he can't breathe freely around her. This is not her fault. He's simply not getting enough time with his male friends.

15. Look to Caring for Children, the Needy, or Animals

We all have the need to give and receive unconditional love and support. When we give unconditionally, it reminds us that we have a place in this world and that we make a difference. Ultimately we are all here to serve each other in love and fairness, yet this truth is often lost or forgotten amid the stresses of life. Our challenge is to integrate giving into our lives to the best of our ability.

Giving unconditionally is easiest when we are giving to those who need us the most and who have little to give back. By caring for children, the poor, or even a pet, we not only help those in need of what we have to offer, we also get to experience the joy of giving without strings attached.

> Giving unconditionally is easiest when we are giving to those who need us the most.

One of the reasons a relationship is so wonderful in the beginning is the lack of strings. We are giving freely, because we assume it will all come back. When, as time goes on, it doesn't come back the way we think it should, then we begin to hold back with our partner or resent him or her for giving less back to us. In a way, we should thank our partner for revealing how conditional our love is, but instead we feel hurt. At these times, the real source of our pain is that we have stopped freely giving the love in our hearts. Our love has ceased to be unconditional.

By taking the time to give unconditionally to those who cannot give back, we remind ourselves of the joy of unconditional giving.

We return to our sense of fullness and are once again willing to let our hearts overflow into our relationship and our life.

16. Look to Books, Movies, Theater and TV

Reading, watching TV or going to the movies or the theater can be great sources of newness. Making sure we take the time to get the stimulation and entertainment we need frees us from expecting our partners to entertain us. A good action or adventure movie can stimulate a lot of testosterone for a man. Likewise a romantic drama or "chick flick" can do wonders to raise a woman's oxytocin levels. Having a good book to stretch out with can also be a great stimulator of heavenly hormones for either sex.

Our lives are enriched by others' experiences.

But another value in books, movies, theater, and TV is hearing stories from other people's lives. This, in turn, increases our awareness of the stories in our own lives. Soon we find ourselves sharing things with our partners that would never have come up if someone else's story hadn't prompted the sharing.

17. Look to What We Eat and How We Exercise

We have already explored in great detail the importance of good food and regular exercise. Without implementing a healthy diet or food plan and including plenty of walking or exercise, many people experience mood swings, anxiety, and depression to various degrees. Research shows that proper exercise alone is more effective than any antidepressant. Even moderate exercise a few hours a week can help us feel good about ourselves. The endorphins produced by exercise not only take away physical pain, but they also increase self-esteem.

Our ability to give and receive love is greatly diminished when we are not feeling our best much of the time. Understanding the importance of superfoods and the blood sugar-stabilizing contribution of PGX® makes a huge difference in our individual health and the quality of our shared relationships. Improving the quality of our relationships doesn't necessarily mean loving our partner more; it just means we have the energy to share our health and happiness with the person we love.

Research shows that exercise alone can be more effective than any anti-depressant.

Just cutting down on processed foods can reduce fatigue and stress in a matter of days. Using superminerals to support optimal brain function boosts healthy brain chemicals like dopamine and serotonin. As long as we are lacking the nutrition we need, we will always feel like something is missing in our love relationship.

18. Look to Your Sleep Requirements

People often deprive themselves of sleep in order to get more done. However, they fail to realize that by getting better sleep, stress levels decrease and they can get more done in less time. As lack of sleep causes our stress levels to increase, this, in turn, prevents us from sleeping deeply. Making sleep a priority will give you the support you need to start each day with renewed energy and optimism.

Sleep well and you will start each day with renewed optimism.

A good night's sleep allows you to let go of the frustrations, disappointments and concerns of the day. If you are worried or frustrated in the evening, rather than venting to your partner about it and ruining his or her sleep, go to bed and let your brain process it for you. In the morning it will no longer seem such a big deal. It will be easier to let it go.

Often I see couples drag their relationship down by talking too much about their individual feelings of frustration and disappointment. By getting enough sleep, the need to think and talk too much about problems disappears. When there is stress in our lives, chances are, we need more sleep.

Making Your Dreams Come True

By taking the time to nurture your many non-relationship needs, you are not only creating the life you were born to live, you are increasing the joy and satisfaction that that comes from giving freely to your partner. With a full tank of outside love and stimulation, you experience the wonderful feeling of having more to give instead of feeling like you're running on empty all the time.

Finding love in all the right places is one of the best strategies I know to help couples make their dreams come true. But this strategy can backfire if you don't adopt it with the correct attitude. If you take time to get love and support from people and places, but without the right attitude, you may use it against yourself and your relationship. Here are few examples of how we mishandle the support we get in life, and limit the production of our feel-good hormones:

"My friend accepts me just the way I am, why can't you?"

"This is a wonderful vacation; if only my partner would have come so that we could have enjoyed it together."

"Why don't you understand me? Everyone in my support group does."

"Everyone at work thinks I am brilliant; why don't you?"

"I enjoy gardening; I wish my partner loved it as much as I do."

"My partner doesn't like action movies so she stayed home."

"Carol's husband is a cook. I wish my partner would at least help out in the kitchen."

"The farmers market is such a wonderful community experience. If only my partner would share it with me. I don't like going alone."

"I had such a good time at dancing class. But I don't know why I bother: my husband just sits in front of the television."

"What a beautiful sunset! Too bad my partner's busy making calls."

"Look at that loving couple over by the bandstand. I remember when my partner used to hold me that way."

In each of these examples we are focusing on what we are not getting from our partner and thus minimizing the support available to us from other sources. Instead of feeling gratitude and fulfillment for the love we are getting "from all the right places," we use it to justify our feelings of victimhood. Instead of having more to bring home to our romantic partner, we have less. This is what's too often clear: In some ways, the more we get from the world, the more we resent that our partner can't or won't provide that same kind of support.

It is unhealthy to expect our partner to be just like us. If that were true, where would we find the newness that keeps a relationship vital? Shared likes and dislikes are comforting, but too much sameness creates boredom. It's the differences between people that create attraction and passion.

When we stop expecting our partners to be like us, think like us, and make us feel good, and choose instead to take that responsibility upon ourselves, we automatically have more we can give our partners. Even better, they will have so much more to give back to us! Nobody likes to feel they owe someone something, especially something as big as happiness. Feelings of obligation kill romance just as easily as they ruin friendships.

How about looking at things differently? Try saying, "If my partner doesn't like to dance, then I ought to appreciate that I have friends who do like to dance." Such a shift in perspective can change your life. Indeed, it's the basis for making all your dreams come true. We all deserve so much more than we get from the world—that's just how life is. Our job is to open our hearts to recognize where we can get the support we need, and go after it!

Realizing what is Most Important

What does it take to wake us up to what is important in life? Is it the familiar name on the obituary page of the newspaper? Is it the close call in the car? Or the natural disaster that occurred in the city your beloved was visiting?

When we feel this close to losing someone, things suddenly become clear. And, at the top of the list of what matters is loving and being loved. When life looks like it may be about to end, whether it's our life or the life of someone close to us, we reflect on the quality of our close relationships. Our greatest joys and sorrows come from the experiences we have, and the decisions we make, in regard to our intimate partnerships.

To me, the most obvious symptom of our society's increasing stress is our tendency to disregard what is most important in life. Having time to love our partner and others close to us is one of the greatest gifts in life, and yet we often do not realize this until it is too late and the opportunity is gone.

I hear the same story repeatedly from heart disease and cancer survivors. They suddenly realize that their priorities in life were wrong. They made money, and success became more important to them than simply having time to love the people close to them. They failed to immerse themselves in the joy that each day brings. After the threat to their survival subsided, they reduced the demands they were making on life and themselves. They came to appreciate just being alive.

Unfortunately, these people had to suffer greatly before they reached this realization. But we don't need to have a near-death experience to learn this lesson. If we learn how to lower our stress, we can dispel the illusion that we don't have the time or energy to love and cherish the people who are most important to us.

Heart disease and cancer survivors often re-prioritize their lives.

We need to learn to see the forest for the trees. A man will give his heart and soul to make enough money to provide for his family, and then come home too tired to even talk with them. Likewise, a woman will give with all her heart to support her husband and children—and then resent them for not giving back the kind of support she herself thrives on giving. Under the influence of stress, both men and women forget why all humans of both genders do what they do.

Women love to give. They do not give to get back. That is the joy in caring for someone. But when stress takes hold and her hormones run low, a woman forgets that she is doing what nourishes her soul. Instead of freely giving, she starts to resent doing the things she used to love doing. There is no greater pleasure than giving selflessly to someone you love, but unfortunately, this pleasure becomes diminished when a person is overwhelmed by stress.

Men love to give, too. Men happily endure the hardships and sacrifices required to succeed in the work world, and they do it simply to provide for their loved ones. Without someone to love or a family to care for, a man's life is empty. To protect and serve his wife and family is what gives his life meaning and purpose. So, if and when his woman gives him messages that he is not doing enough, his heart is broken and turns to ice. The change is often so gradual that he doesn't even know that it has happened. Just as a woman's role in life has expanded to include work outside the home, so has a man's role expanded beyond merely providing. Now he must also offer emotional support to help his wife cope with the new stresses in her life.

However, the new kind of support that women need from men can only be effective when both partners first take responsibility for their well-being. To manifest our vision of what we can create in our love relationship, we must first learn to balance our hormones and feel good again, regardless of how our partner behaves or responds. By restoring our heavenly hormone levels and feeling good through our own efforts, we can then look once again to our partner, our relationships and our life as an opportunity to give rather than receive.

> To protect and serve his wife and family gives a man's life meaning and purpose.

We also need to take off our rose-colored glasses and see our partners as they are, not as we would wish them to be. While it may seem unromantic to give up expecting your partner to be perfect, it is actually quite the opposite. There is nothing more wonderful and romantic than to fully love someone, faults and all. No one is perfect, and to be fully loved in spite of our imperfections is a blessing that some people only dream of. Learning to feel and express real love is—or ought to be—the apex of any relationship.

Similarly, we need to accept that our love is strongest when it is buttressed by the love and support each partner receives outside the relationship. Giving up on making your partner the only source of love is one of the smartest decisions you will ever make. It is not, as some would think, a defeatist idea. Adjusting our expectations does not mean we are settling for a relationship that doesn't give us everything we want and need. Instead, it is a realistic and healthy approach that almost all happily married couples learn to adopt in some way.

> Adjusting our expectations does not mean we are settling for less.

By committing ourselves to getting the love and support we need in life without putting the burden solely on the back of a romantic partner, we actually release the hormones that renew our romance again and again. Whenever you feel like you are missing something in your relationship, take a moment to reflect on how happy you are. Take responsibility for feeling really good, because then it will be easy for your partner to go that last 10 percent toward making you feel great.

Finding our Way in Life

Life is a process of gradually discovering that we have everything we need—and we always did. I want to tell you a story that illustrates my point.

I knew a man who lived to help other people. He gave time and money to a variety of charities and, as he showed me the sports club he had built in the slums of Houston, I marveled at the many people who came up to greet him by name and shake his hand. But one day, he disappeared—he just never came home. A day or two later, his car was found and police made the gruesome discovery of his body in the trunk. He had been robbed, apparently by one of the many hitchhikers he had picked up to help over the years. His assailant took his wallet, locked him into the trunk of the car and left him for dead.

Despite heat and humidity, he lived for hours, maybe many hours. I later saw how he had unscrewed a tail light to get fresh air, and how he had battered at the underside of the trunk with a screwdriver hoping that someone might hear him and rescue him.

Still, the most unfortunate part of the story was the one I learned myself, after lowering my own body into the trunk of that very same car. The button he would have needed to pop the trunk was within reach! With some coaching from people standing on the outside, I found I could open it myself, simply by sticking my hand out through the tail light, twisting it a little bit to the left, and stretching out my fingers. It wasn't easy, but it wasn't difficult either. After a couple of tries, I could pop that trunk in little more than a second. I wondered, if I can do it, why couldn't he? All I can assume is that he didn't know it was possible. There was no one outside that day, no one who could tell him what they could see and he could not.

The man who died trapped in that trunk was my father. I miss him greatly.

In some ways, I consider my father's death an allegory for the purpose of my life and teachings. I am committed to answering the questions people have about their relationships and their health. I try to show them how to escape from whatever "trunk" they may be trapped in. I try to provide the outside perspective that my father didn't have.

I hope that by reading this book, you have discovered some of the "buttons" in your life, and that your new insights will allow you to unlock whatever trunk may be confining you in your life or your love. Don't stop trying. Stretch a little further. Whatever you're hoping to find is well within your reach. Remember: You have everything you need, and you always did.

VENUS ON FIRE MARS ON ICE

There are times when simply opening an email can provide me with boundless hope for the future. Here's a story that came to me from a woman in Florida. Only the names have been changed.

"While driving with my two grandkids, James, 8, and Emma, 4, I heard them arguing, with Emma complaining and James being passive-aggressive. This wasn't unusual behavior for these two, but it struck me that they sounded very Venus-and-Mars. So I decided to try a little John Gray on them.

"I said, 'Let's have a sweetness contest. Emma, you start by very sweetly asking James if he can find that toy you dropped. Tell him how much it would help you if he finds it.' She did that very well. James found the toy and gave it to her. 'Great,' I said. 'Now tell him how much you appreciate what he did.' She did, with great enthusiasm, and he seemed pleased... and very glad that she had stopped complaining!

"I said, 'James, is there a nice compliment you could give your sister?' This didn't come easily. 'Something about her that's special?' After a few attempts, he came up with, 'Emma, your hair is really long and you look kind of like the pictures in your princess books.' This delighted her and she went on and on about princesses. 'Be sure to thank him for that nice compliment,' I said. She did, and they began trading compliments and thank yous to see who could be the sweetest. When they got out of the car, Emma ran over to hug him and said, 'I love you, James!'

"How amazing that this simple little step that John prescribes for adults—asking him politely for what she wants, in his language, and then enthusiastically appreciating him for what he does, followed by him complimenting her for who she is—could have the same effect on little children that it does in adult relationships! To me, this proves that there are natural differences between males and females at any age, and simple little changes can turn relationships from upsetting to loving very quickly. Thank you John Gray!"

No, thank you, I thought to myself as I finished reading. By sharing her gender intelligence with her grandchildren, this woman is doing more than helping them grow up to be wonderful partners to those they choose to love. She is helping them discover patterns of relating that will carry through all they do, reducing their stress and improving their health, maybe even increasing their longevity. In a world where it often seems that we have lost so much—our sense of our selves, our focus on what's important, even our connection to the things that keep us strong and sane— here is proof of what we stand to gain: A better future for us all.

FOR MORE INFORMATION

For more information on the concepts and products presented in this book, visit **BalancedPlanets.com**, or **venus-on-fire-mars-on-ice.com**. You can also call **1-866-573-9362**.

There are many sources of good information available on the natural health supplements and herbs mentioned in this book. In addition to your local health food store, your health care professional, bookstores, and libraries, there are many online sources of information, including the Dietary Supplement Education Alliance website, **www.supplementinfo.org**, the Counsel for Responsible Nutrition's Life. Supplemented website, **www.lifesupplemented.org**, and the American Botanical Association website **www.herbalgram.org**. For information on PGX® (PolyGlycopleX®) visit **www.pgx.com**.

TO FIND A NATURAL HEALTH PRODUCT STORE NEAR YOU

—U.S.A.—

Visit www.naturalfactors.com and click on *"Where to Buy"*

—CANADA—

Visit **www.pno.ca** and click on *"Find a Store"*

Appendix A

CHAPTER 9

One Hundred Oxytocin-Producing Activities A Woman Can Engage In

1. Getting a regular massage
2. Creating a change of pace and feeling pampered by getting your hair done
3. Special "spa time" getting a manicure or pedicure
4. Venus night out (taking time with a support group of women only)
5. Talking on the phone to a friend about personal issues and not just work-related ones
6. Sharing a non-business related meal with friends
7. Preparing for a party and cooking together with friends
8. Cleaning up after a gathering with friends
9. Making it a family project to paint a room
10. Listening to your favorite music
11. Singing out loud in the shower and/or taking singing lessons
12. Singing in a group just for fun
13. Taking a scented bath with soft music and candle light
14. Creating a special occasion by lighting candles at dinner
15. Leisure shopping with a friend who likes to shop
16. Vacationing with girl friends at a spa
17. Taking a low intensity aerobic class without getting out of breath
18. Getting special attention by working out with a personal trainer

19. Joining a Yoga class and not rushing off to work
20. Going out dancing with friends or taking a dancing class.
21. Easy walking for at least an hour while talking with a friend or friends
22. Anticipating a regular walk and talk with special walking buddies
23. Offering to help by preparing meals for friends with new babies
24. Offering unsolicited help by preparing meals for friends and family who are sick
25. After a warm shower finishing with cold water within a comfortable refreshing range. (When nipples become erect it is due to a release of oxytocin)
26. Taking time to smell the roses and other fragrant flowers in the garden
27. Enjoying and arranging fresh cut flowers in the home
28. Growing and tending to a vegetable garden
29. Preparing a meal from your own garden
30. Making a special dish and giving the recipe to your guests
31. Taking walks in nature away from cars and houses
32. Going camping or river rafting with a group
33. Holding a baby
34. Petting, holding and caring for a pet
35. Asking for directions when you need help
36. Asking someone to carry something for you
37. Asking for help even when it is something small but it would make your day easier
38. Browsing in book store with no agenda
39. Reading series of nonfiction books
40. Learning new recipes and sharing them with a friend
41. Taking a cooking class
42. Getting help with cooking, shopping, and house care

43. Hiring a handyman to make your life easier
44. Getting help to plan fun family activities
45. Cooking for special occasions
46. Attending and participating in a parent teacher association meeting
47. Baking and bringing your favorite desserts to be sold or shared at fundraisers
48. Enjoying a vacation on a warm island or breezy mountain top
49. Attending live theater and concerts
50. Getting help from others to plan picnics with friends and family
51. Attending or participating in dance performances
52. Creating special occasions to look forward to
53. Sharing in a new mothers club or babysitting your grandchildren
54. Taking care of children in some capacity for work or for family
55. Finding opportunities to help or feed the hungry
56. Caring for and watering plants and flowers in the garden
57. Reading magazines about fashion and people
58. Attending regular inspirational or spiritual gatherings
59. Keeping in touch with friends by e-mail, phone or cards
60. Watching your favorite TV show with a friend
61. Listening to inspirational tapes or CD's
62. Regular sharing and Venus Talks with a therapist, coach or Mars/Venus telephone coach
63. Learning and practicing a musical instrument
64. Studying about and then visiting a new culture with a friend
65. Spending time at the beach, a river or a lake
66. Meeting together with friends after a day of recreation

67. Enjoying wine tasting with friends
68. Peacefully demonstrating for a social or political cause
69. Going to or participating in a local parade
70. Hiring someone to help you clean house and remove the clutter
71. Offering to help a friend paint a room or work in their garden
72. Taking a class in nutrition or wellness
73. Reading poetry, writing poetry or going to a poetry reading
74. Visiting and touring an art or museum exhibit
75. Listening to an author speak at the local bookstore or library
76. Keeping a journal of your daily thoughts and feelings
77. Keeping a photo journal for each of your children
78. Creating an email list of friends so that you can easily send them recent photos and get theirs
79. Creating an email list of friends with like political views to give your support and receive theirs
80. Taking a class with a friend on painting or sculpture
81. Sharing an espresso or tea with friends
82. Making a charitable donation
83. Getting a sun tan
84. Changing your hair color
85. Buying a new outfit
86. Shopping for sexy lingerie
87. Renting and watching a romantic movie
88. Sharing a picture album with friends
89. Changing the wall color in your home and painting it yourself
90. Learning and practicing a new diet plan for better health
91. Donating your older clothes to a charity
92. Preparing a will for your children or friends

93. Driving a car that is good for the environment
94. Making artistic fruit arrangements in your kitchen.
95. Preparing a special meal for a friend using your best silver, plates and napkins
96. Getting all dressed up and going out with your girl friends
97. Taking a class on flower arrangements for the home
98. Baking a cake to bring to a party or as a hostess gift
99. Asking a friend to give you a birthday party
100. Volunteering at a local hospital or hospice to help the old and dying

Appendix B

CHAPTER 11

Grounded to the Earth

It is well-established, though not widely known, that the surface of the earth possesses a limitless and continuously renewed supply of free or mobile electrons. Any conductive object, coupled with the earth, will immediately conduct earth's free electrons and equalize with them and thereafter maintain the charge of the earth. Human and animal bodies are conductive and when they are coupled with the earth, they also conduct and become saturated with the earth's mobile electrons.

Connecting with a steady supply of the earth's electrons is not only something people have done for thousands of years, but it has amazing benefits. Have you ever noticed how good you feel while walking barefoot on the beach or swimming in the ocean or a pool? Clinton observed that after about 40 minutes of direct contact with the earth or the ocean much of the pain in your body temporarily disappears.

With regular contact with the earth, the results of decreased inflammation become more permanent. This natural process of connecting to the earth he calls grounding. With direct skin to earth contact or through some conductive substance, million of electrons flow into the body neutralizing free radicals, minimizing inflammation. Unfortunately, when we wear shoes with rubber soles we are not connected to the earth.

For thousands of years, people have gone barefoot or they have used leather soles for walking. In just the last 50 years we have changed from leather soles to rubber soles. Leather soles conduct the earth's electrons while rubber soles do not. Rubber soles completely insulate us from the earth's natural beneficial EMF field. It is no coincidence that in the last 50 years, the incidence of inflammatory diseases has dramatically increased along with record levels of sleep problems.

Using thermal images, Clinton proved that grounding dramatically reduced inflammation in only 40 minutes. As inflammation disappeared, pain also disappeared. Grounding is not only good for pain relief but, by decreasing inflammation, it promotes faster wound healing. In addition, it lowers cortisol levels at night, thus improving sleep.

These results of improved sleep, as reported by members of one of America's winning bicycle teams, have been borne out in sleep studies. When sleeping on sheets that are grounded, cortisol levels in every participant would begin to normalize and synchronize with normal circadian rhythms so that cortisol levels would reach their lowest levels around midnight. This normalization of cortisol rhythms not only improves sleep, but allows deep sleep to last longer.

As we have already explored, longer deep sleep releases more growth hormone which promotes regeneration and rejuvenation of the mind and body. Deep sleep normalizes adrenal function, resulting in healthy hormone production. A good night's sleep is the foundation for creating the hormones of love, desire, and longevity.

Staying grounded while sleeping at night minimizes the effects of EMFs.

The public today is gradually hearing more about the unhealthy effects of EMFs (electromagnetic frequencies). The question being debated today is not if it is bad, but simply how much of it will do real and lasting damage. It is one thing to be several feet away from a source of unhealthy frequencies. It is quite another to put the source against your head for a long period time as in the case of cell phones.

Some claim that extended exposure to electromagnetic fields (EMF) from power lines, home wiring, airport and military radar, substations, transformers, computers and appliances can cause brain tumors, leukemia, birth defects, miscarriages, chronic fatigue, headaches, cataracts, heart problems, stress, nausea, chest pain, forgetfulness, cancer and other health problems. Hundreds of studies on this subject have produced contradictory results, yet some experts are convinced that the threat is real.

Dr. David Carpenter, Dean at the School of Public Health, State University of New York believes it is likely that up to 30% of all childhood cancers come from exposure to EMFs. With increasing research at the most prestigious universities, protecting ourselves from harmful EMFs is no longer some kooky concern. Even the Environmental Protection Agency (EPA) warns, "There is reason for concern" and advises "prudent avoidance". I know for some people this seems "too far out," but consider how many years we knew that cigarette smoking causes cancer before it became mainstream. Yet even today one of the biggest causes of death is cigarettes.

If you wish to follow the EPA's advice and practice "prudent avoidance," then here are a few helpful suggestions.

Measure your home, work and school environments with a Gauss meter. Gauss meters are inexpensive and can easily be ordered on the internet from a variety of catalogs and sites. The EPA has proposed a safety standard of 1 mG. However, many experts believe we should maintain our own living and sleeping quarters at 0.5 mG and below.

Measure EMFs both inside and outside your home. Don't let your children play near power lines, transformers, radar domes and microwave towers. Avoid areas where the field is above 1 mG.

Measure the EMFs from appliances both when they are operating and when they are turned off. Some appliances (like TVs) are still drawing current even when they are off. Don't sit too close to your TV set. Distance yourself at least 6 feet away. Use a Gauss meter to help you decide where it is safe to sit. Fortunately, the new flat screen TV's put out much less EMFs than the old tube TVs.

Don't sleep under an electric blanket or on a waterbed. If you insist on using these, unplug them before going to bed (don't just turn it off). Even though there is no magnetic field when they are turned off, there may still be a high electric field.

Rearrange your office and home area so that you are not exposed to EMFs from the sides and backs of electric appliances and computers. In the home, it is best that all major electrical appliances, such as computers, TVs, refrigerators etc, be placed up against outside walls. That way you are not creating an EMF field in the adjoining room.

Don't sit too close to your computer. Computer monitors vary greatly in the strength of their EMFs, so you should check yours with a meter. Don't stand close to or in front of your microwave oven when it is on. (Ideally, get rid of it. Radiating your food is not a good idea either)

Eyeglass frames should ideally be made from plastic with no wires in them, otherwise they can serve as an antenna to focus the radio and cellular phone waves directly into your brain.

Be wary of cordless appliances such as electric toothbrushes and razors. Avoid wearing watches with batteries. And last, but not least, always remember that EMFs pass right through walls. The EMF you are reading on your Gauss meter could be radiating from the next room... or from outside your home.

Move all electrical appliances at least 6 feet from your bed. Eliminate wires running under your bed. Unfortunately it is much more difficult to eliminate or move electric wires within the walls.

These wires can be easily shielded, but home builders rarely do. These wires are generally at about three feet high, around the same level where our head rests while sleeping at night. This exposure is not a good idea. These EMF radiations can be avoided if builders put them in an insulating tube. It is a federal requirement that all hospitals, schools and public buildings have this shielding around electric wires, but it is a not yet a requirement in homes.

One of the other measureable problems with unhealthy EMFs is that it immediately reduces your body's zeta potential. By reducing our exposure to harmful EMFs, you can witness the change under the microscope. With high EMF exposure blood cells become sluggish and congested. After just 30 minutes of touching the earth with your bare feet the zeta potential goes up in your body and your bloods cells separate leaving them plump and round ready to absorb more oxygen and remove toxins. When I heard about this research I went out and bought an expensive microscope to test this. I saw this with my own eyes.

Electricity is an inseparable part of our modern day society and will continue to be all around us. Most experts agree that limited, non-chronic exposure to EMFs is not a threat. Minimizing exposure to electricity is good, but what is still missing from this conversation is the importance of taking time to activate and ground your cells in a non electric field, i.e. nature.

Humans and animals have lived in conductive (barefoot) contact with the earth for thousands of years. With the introduction of plastic and other materials that insulate us from the earth, we have unknowing cut ourselves off from the benefits of the earth's electromagnetic field. At the same time we have increased our exposure to the harmful effects of high frequency electric fields. While there are many reasons for the dramatic decreases in hormone production found around the world in just the last 30 years, a lack of grounding may prove to be one of the most significant reasons. By grounding ourselves and creating better sleep routines we are insuring an abundance of healthy hormone production.

Sleeping on these sheets not only provides the negative ions from the earth to neutralise free radical damage in your body, but also protects you from any unhealthy EMFs in your bedroom. You can find out more about grounding products at BalancedPlanets.com.

Appendix C

CHAPTER 12

Herbal Supplements for Increased Sexual Desire and Enhanced Performance

For Both Men and Women:

1. *Epimedium* (horny goat weed) helps increase sexual desire as well as provides extra stamina. It was discovered in ancient China when goat herders noticed that on certain hills where this weed grew wild, the goats were sexually active all day long and hence the name horny goat weed. Research in China has demonstrated that taking supplements of epimedium can lower cortisol levels. This stress-lowering benefit is an extra bonus and probably a big reason why it can be so helpful in the bedroom.

2. *Eurycoma Longfolia* (tongkat Ali) for one of the most powerful of all sexual performance enhancers for men and for women. It has been used for over a thousand years in Malaysia for sexual rejuvenation and performance. This herb can help a man sustain his erection for as long as is needed to provide a woman with maximum pleasure.

3. *Tribulus Terrestros* has been used in Asia and Bulgaria for years to treat libido and infertility problems. With regular use it has a powerful ability to increase testosterone levels and as a result increase sexual desire, hardness of erections and stamina. In one study testosterone levels increased by 41%. Besides lowering stress levels for men, testosterone generates sexual desire in both men and women.

4. **Maca** is not only a superfood for stimulating hormone production, but is also well-known for its ability to enhance libido. People in Peru have been eating maca roots for centuries to enhance fertility and sexual performance in both sexes. It helps increase sexual stamina in men and sexual interest and responsiveness in women.

5. **Yohimbi bark** has one of the strongest reputations for increasing sexual activity in both men and women. One must be careful not to take more than is recommended. In this case, "more" is not better. If one has high blood pressure or experiences heart palpitations then it is not recommended at all. It is a powerful blood dilator increasing blood flow to the genitals and has been shown in human studies at National Institute of Health to be effective in the treatment of male impotence.

6. *Avena Sativa* (wild oats) is known to awaken a woman's interest in having sex while it has the effect of slowing down a man's need to ejaculate. While this doesn't stimulate a man's desire it does help him to last longer.

7. **Muira Puama** (potency wood) is known in South American to provide increased sexual potency. It has been used as therapy for both fatigue and impotency.

8. **Saw Palmetto** can help promote sexual health for both men and woman's sexual functions. It helps to rejuvenate her reproductive organs. In addition it is widely known to assist in reducing the swelling of the male prostate gland.

9. **Ashwaganda** is a herb from India known for its ability to enhance sex by stimulating dopamine and serotonin in the brain. It is also a powerful adaptogen known to assist the body in coping effectively with stress.

Additional Herbs for Women:

10. **Kacip fatima** is a performance-enhancing herb from Malaysia particularly known for its ability to increase pleasure for women. By increasing blood flow to her clitoris and natural lubrication in her vagina it enhances the pleasure of sexual stimulation. Kacip fatima should not be used by pregnant women as it has also been, for centuries to induce labor. Just as oxytocin induces labor in women, it also activates her sexual responses. It may be that Kacip fatima increases a woman's sexual responses by helping to raise her oxytocin levels.

11. **Licorice** contains an estrogenic activity that can increase a woman's ability to utilize oxytocin to increase her sexual response and more easily achieve orgasm.

12. **Damiana** is an aphrodisiac from Mexico known to help stimulate sexual feelings particularly in women. It has also been used for asthma, anxiety, depression, headache, and menstrual disorders. Each of these conditions has been known to prevent a woman's arousal. By helping the body deal with these symptoms, she is better able to enjoy sex.

Functional Chocolates for Romance

The following is a brief description of the benefits of each of the added amino acids:

1. **Theanine** helps to calm the brain without sedating it. It does this by activating GABA levels which calm us while also stimulating dopamine levels which excite us.

2. **GABA** has a calming effect in the brain very similar to the benefits we have already discussed regarding Theanine. It helps slow the process down allowing us to enjoy each moment more.

3. **Glycine** is added to the mixture because it has been known to enhance the effects of GABA as well, assist the body in sustaining healthy blood sugar levels. When we are under stress the body uses up it's supply of glycine very quickly. Taking glycine can help sustain a steady supply of fuel to the brain.

4. **Taurine** is an amino acid which is now being used in a lot of caffeinated energy drinks. It is used because it has the ability to help the brain sustain dopamine levels. Dopamine is one of the main romantic hormones.

5. **5-HTP** is an amino acid extracted from the graffonia seed that converts into serotonin. Serotonin is the feel good brain chemical allowing us to forget our worries and appreciate what we have.

6. **Guarana** helps by stimulating dopamine levels. Dopamine is the pleasure hormones which motivates and excites us. Used together with chocolate, these natural ingredients become a potent Mars-Venus romantic love potion.

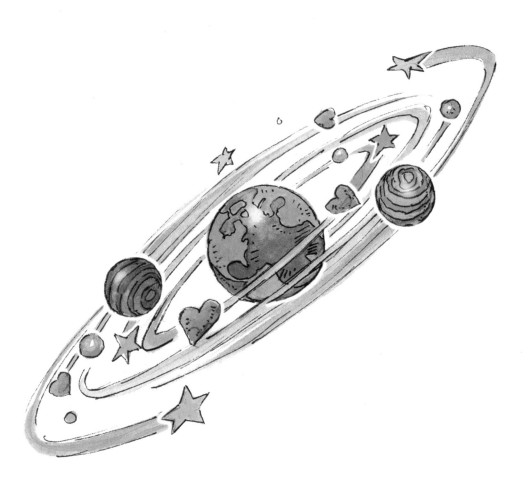

BalancedPlanets.com